WITHDRAWN

HEALTH CARE IN TRANSITION

LEARNING CLINICAL SKILLS

PEARLS, PITFALLS AND TIPS FOR THE OSCE

HEALTH CARE IN TRANSITION

Additional books in this series can be found on Nova's website under the Series tab.

Additional E-books in this series can be found on Nova's website under the E-book tab.

HEALTH CARE IN TRANSITION

LEARNING CLINICAL SKILLS

PEARLS, PITFALLS AND TIPS FOR THE OSCE

BRIDGET MAHER
AND
PAT HENN
EDITORS

Nova Science Publishers, Inc.
New York

For permission to use material from this book please contact us:
Telephone 631-231-7269; Fax 631-231-8175
Web Site: http://www.novapublishers.com

Additional color graphics may be available in the e-book version of this book.

LIBRARY OF CONGRESS CATALOGING-IN-PUBLICATION DATA
Learning clinical skills : pearls, pitfalls, and tips for the OSCE / editors, Bridget Maher and Pat Henn.
p. ; cm.
Includes bibliographical references and index.
ISBN 978-1-62100-409-7 (hardcover)
I. Maher, Bridget. II. Henn, Pat.
[DNLM: 1. Clinical Competence--Case Reports. 2. Clinical Medicine--education--Case Reports. 3. Students, Medical--Case Reports. W 21.5]
LC classification not assigned
616--dc23
2011034206

Published by Nova Science Publishers, Inc. † New York

Contents

Preface

Listening to the patient's story, asking the right questions, and doing a careful, thorough and informed physical examination are intrinsic to good medicine. It is easy to rely on and become dependant on technology to diagnose and to treat our patients. Yet no machine will ever be a match for a listening ear and the laying on of hands. These skills are core to the Art of Medicine and need practice. It is only by becoming familiar with the norm that we can appreciate the abnormal. This textbook is a clinical skills textbook with a third dimension – the human factor. We read about real people, real symptoms and real diagnostic problems. The book doesn't waste time on rare physical signs but focuses on common, important clinical skills and symptom patterns. Medical students cannot expect to be expert diagnosticians – this only comes with experience. But they can learn how to take a careful history, how to do a thorough physical examination and how to put it all together.

For centuries, doctors have practiced examination skills that when properly performed, offer a wealth of information. In this textbook, medical experts share their wisdom, their advice and their experiences. The book is patient-focused, as medicine is. After describing a clinical case, the authors discuss the case, using it to give advice on history-taking skills, physical examination techniques and suggested investigations. We are given the 'pearls' or key nuggets of information: we are given the pitfalls – the frequently commited errors, the easy to make mistakes, and we are given what lies close to every student's heart – tips for the OSCE examination. Each chapter also has a 'Lab-Spot' which focuses on relevant important laboratory investigations.

In planning this book, we did something that few other textbooks have done – we asked our medical students what they wanted from a medical textbook, what topics they would like to see covered and what were the areas that they found particularly difficult. The result is a very practical, hands-on, patient-focused clinical textbook, which, while not covering every single topic, manages to cover the important things; common, everyday things like dyspnoea and fainting, diarrhoea and diabetes.

This is what real medicine is about – taking a good history, doing a good clinical examination and making the right call. This requires highly-developed diagnostic, communication and problem-solving skills.

We are all aware of the heavy workload of medical students and doctors in training. This is why we wanted a clinical skills book that was user-friendly and accessible, with lots of tables, lists and practice points. We hope that 'Pearls and Pitfalls' will continue to be used by students after they qualify. This is a book not confined by technological and laboratory advances; it is dateless and timeless because it is based on honing and fine-tuning those very skills that doctors have practiced for centuries and will continue to practice.

This book is written by clinicians who have a passion for teaching, who are enthusiastic about passing on their wisdom, and who take joy from the practice of medicine. These qualities emanate from this textbook – along with energy, positivity and humanity. These clinicians are giving that very precious gift – their own experience of the Science and Art of Medicine. We send them our warmest thanks.

Introduction

All medical students and doctors in training search for the "magic" clinical textbook. Such a tome would contain lists which prompt the correct conclusion, pictures which distil in an image all pertinent clinical features of a condition whilst also conveying the wisdom of the experts who often have lifelong clinical experience in the areas about which they write. Drs Maher and Henn, who are experienced in Medical Education, have never found such a textbook, nor have I.

There are, of course, a range of clinical handbooks and textbooks pitched at undergraduate medical students or doctors in the early years of training. The approach usually adopted is a comprehensive list of questions which must be asked in the history; a list of symptoms and signs layered with current knowledge. Students and trainees, however, really want to know how the expert approaches the typical case. They look for a tool which opens the door into the mindset and the wisdom acquired over years. When is a cough something to worry about? How do they manage to evaluate a patient with diarrhoea in minutes? What lists do senior doctors really use?

Drs Maher and Henn evaluated all the clinical textbooks available and clearly have identified a gap in the market. *'Learning Clinical Skills –Pearls, Pitfalls and Tips For The OSCE'* is written through the lens of a student by experts in each of the topics who have extensive experience in teaching both undergraduate medical students and specialist trainees. All contributors were asked to identify exemplar clinical cases which represent a typical undifferentiated patient presentation, reflect on the issues students find challenging when interpreting such presentations, honestly declare any mistakes that they, the experts, themselves occasionally make, whilst also reviewing some of the key diagnostic tests and noting the limitations of such investigations.

The 'Pearls' in these chapters capture the golden nuggets or key teaching events which all doctors in training encounter when in the presence of good mentors and teachers. These are the moments when "it all comes together" for a student because the expert leads the trainee through the steps they themselves take in navigating the presentation and consultation. System by system, a conversational and frequently humorous approach is adopted, leading the reader through the scenarios and sequences of decisions to be made before reaching a conclusion.

The 'Pitfalls' are the common mistakes that the contributors themselves have either made or observed, in practice over the years. While no text can replace the one-to-one mentorship and apprenticeship of good clinical training, the "it happened to me" sections certainly have a high impact. Clinicians describe a near miss or a time where they could have got it wrong. We tell our students that "to err is human", yet we rarely, if ever, share our own failings with them and certainly few texts ever acknowledge these. All clinicians are as influenced by their 'near misses' as their successes. This is a more honest clinical text which notes the uncertainty of clinical practice and tries to reveal the real guiding principles many of us adhere to on a day-to-day basis.

On reading the book, one hears the expert talking to the student through the pages. This textbook is not an inert catalogue of lists, nor does it purport to be a comprehensive guide to the entire knowledge base required in medicine. It does, however, focus the student on the approach which should be adopted when encountering common clinical presentations in the young and old. Despite its comparatively short length, any student familiar with this text will emerge with a very sound knowledge base.

Cognisant of the fact that assessment drives all learning, each chapter has handy tips for the representative clinical questions students and trainees are likely to asked in their exams, be they OSCES, long cases or short cases.

Drs Maher and Henn have produced the kind of textbook I wish I had had as a medical student.

In: Learning Clinical Skills
Editors: Bridget Maher and Pat Henn
ISBN: 978-1-62100-409-7

Chapter I

The Consultation

Joe Moran

The relationship between doctors and patients is a dynamic and constantly evolving phenomenon. The dynamics of this relationship are played out in the consultation. The consultation between the patient and doctor (or student) is the basic unit of medical practice. The decisions that arise from this process inform the future care of the patient. It follows that the quality of this process determines the quality and effectiveness of the care provided to the patient. This may sound overly simplistic. However, it is only in relatively recent times that the "consultation" itself has received serious attention from undergraduate medical educators. A number of models of the consultation have been described over the years. These models encourage the doctor to think beyond the purely biological and to include psychological and social dimensions when treating patients. [1]

This expanded function of the consultation is in contrast to the previous model where the emphasis was on "history taking and physical examination". In the "history taking and physical examination" model, the emphasis is primarily biomedical. This concept is being gradually replaced by the biopsychosocial model of care, which puts increased emphasis on the patient's fears and expectations (the patient's agenda). The consultation process itself, when used in this way, possesses an inherent therapeutic value.

This newer biopsychosocial approach serves as a useful model for both teaching and learning modern consultation skills. In summary, medical students need to be aware that an excessive focus on "getting a history from a patient" is poor practice. Alternatively, students need to work on a more patient-centered approach that takes the patient's agenda into account. The medical school at University College Cork, having examined the various models of the consultation that are available, has decided to use the 'Four Habits' (4H) model to teach consultation skills.

Four Habits Model

- Invest in the beginning of the consultation
- Determine the patient's reasons for attending
- Demonstrate empathy
- Invest in the end of the consultation

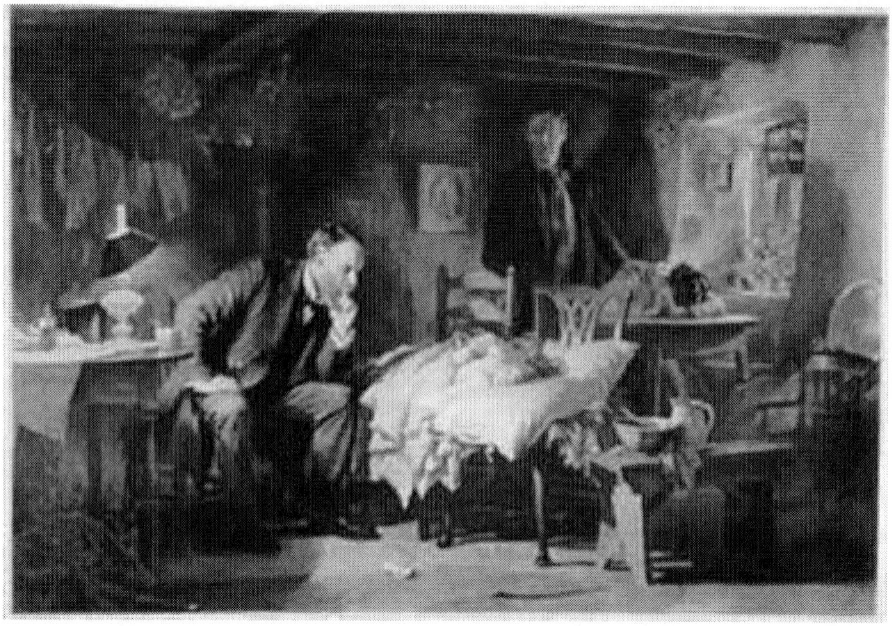

Figure 1. *The Doctor* by Sir Luke Fildes.

This model was chosen because it is evidence-based, pragmatic and of proven acceptability to both patients and doctors in every-day clinical encounters. We intend to help our students become more clinically effective, empathic and safer doctors by teaching them a valid and reliable method of conducting their consultations. Our chosen model is a balanced method that integrates biomedicine with psychological and social medicine. We all want to be better doctors. We believe that the principles outlined are applicable to all medical disciplines and that contrary to popular medical myth, they are not the sole preserve of GPs. General practice has been involved in the evolution of thinking concerning the dynamics of the consultation but it is, in my view, a serious mistake to suggest that these concepts are in any way discipline-specific. Given that there has been a tendency in medical schools to delegate the teaching of this subject to Departments of General Practice or Social Science, it is understandable how this myth arose in the first place. In brief, we believe that the ability to consult effectively with a patient is a core medical skill that every doctor should possess. We reject the Sir Lancelot or Dr House stereotypes that suggest deficiencies in communication skills can be compensated for by the possession of more comprehensive core medical knowledge or procedural skills.

One of the paradoxes of modern medical practice is that while individual patient outcomes have never been better e.g. improved maternal mortality rates, improved cardiovascular disease outcomes, at the same time there has been a rise in patient dissatisfaction with the medical profession in general. Litigation rates and costs have risen and medical malpractice insurance costs are now a significant financial overhead. We believe that the conduct of the consultation has a role in the aetiology of this phenomenon and that improved consultation skills will help both patients and doctors reduce the risks of future litigation.

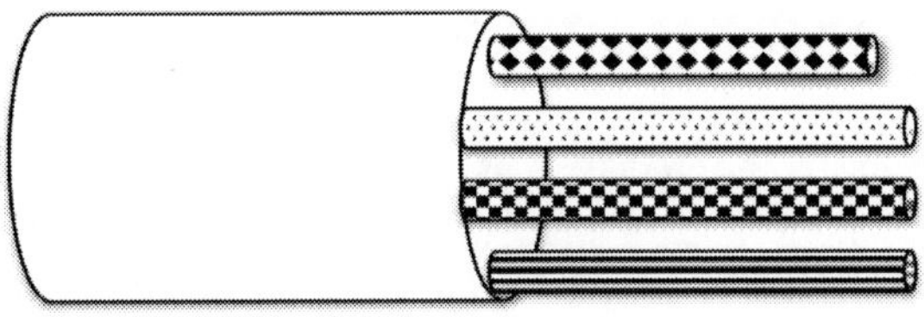

Figure 2. Four Strands of Consultation (image courtesy of Dr Pat Henn).

Practicing doctors need to devote thought as to how they conduct their consultations. Most continuing medical education (CME) and continuing professional development (CPD) activities seem to be devoted to keeping up "to date" with biomedical advances. Learning and honing one's core consultation skills require time on the CME and CPD timetable also. I aim to describe the various components that make up the consultation and demonstrate their respective roles in this introductory chapter.

The consultation is the basic unit or currency of medical practice. It can be likened to a bridge or cable that connects the patient and doctor. Like any structure, it is made up of a series of component parts (strands). In the same way that an electronic cable connects electronic components together, the consultation "connects" the patient and doctor. We all know that electronic cables malfunction when some or all of the component strands are faulty. Similarly, the medical consultation can malfunction if one or more of the consultation strands fail to function properly. This is an important concept to understand.

In this consultation model, there are four strands that need to be functioning properly in order for the consultation to work effectively. These strands are the skills that you will be expected to start to acquire when you begin to meet with patients, either in their homes, the hospital or community-based clinics. These skills or strands are:

- Core Knowledge
- Physical Examination Skills
- Problem-Solving Skills
- Communication Skills.

Core Knowledge

Core knowledge is the basic medical data you have learned to date and will continue to learn for the rest of your career. Initially you acquire this in a didactic manner, mainly by attending lectures. The basic sciences are the main focus initially and as you progress through the course, you are exposed to more clinical patient contact. The emphasis on this form of learning is greatest in the junior undergraduate years. As already mentioned, doctors spend a considerable amount of time and energy working on their core knowledge skills. You can liken this to adding data to your "hard disk". Of interest, when things go wrong clinically it is seldom because of deficits in the doctor's core knowledge. More likely, the cause will be due to a problem in either the doctor's other skills (physical examination, problem solving) or attitudes (communication skills).

Physical Examination Skills

Physical examination skills are easily appreciated as being a core component of the consultation. Students spend a considerable part of their undergraduate and graduate career developing and refining these skills. A major part of your final examinations will be in demonstrating your physical examination abilities e.g. eliciting an ankle reflex, detecting and describing a cardiac murmur. You cannot learn these skills from a book in the library. Rather, they are acquired on the wards and in the clinics. Patient contact is mandatory for these skills to be acquired and developed. Like any other practical skill, it is practice over and over again that leads to mastery in this area. Learning in this area can be supplemented with text-books but they are not a substitute for hands-on experience.

Problem Solving Skills

Problem solving skills are the skills required in order to make "clinical sense" out of the presenting problem(s). You need to integrate the information you have gathered during the consultation, using your core medical knowledge, communication skills and physical examination skills and devise an agreed or negotiated management plan with the patient.

Note that we emphasize the concept of agreeing a management plan with the patient as distinct to simply devising a management plan for the patient. This is a core concept and quite a different way of relating with patients. [2]

Communication Skills

The teaching of communication skills is a relatively new activity for many undergraduate programmes. Frequently it is delegated to Deptartments of General Practice or Social Sciences. There are a few myths concerning communication skills -the main myth being that one is either born a good communicator or not. However, communication skills can be successfully learned and taught. One does not expect students to be born with physical examination skills, and, in our opinion, the same applies to communication skills. These skills need to be clearly articulated and described for the students. Clinicians need to be trained. Students need to see these skills demonstrated by their teachers.

The older autocratic model of the doctor as the one who "knows best" has been replaced by a more balanced model where the patient's agenda is taken into account by the doctor.

Summary

The way in which you conduct your consultations will have a serious bearing on your performance as a clinician. You are more likely to have improved clinical outcomes and less likely to be involved in malpractice complaints if you adopt a patient-centered approach in your consultations. The essential strands of the consultation are core knowledge, physical examination skills, problem-solving skills and communication skills. Proficiency in all four skills is required in order to successfully conduct a patient-centered consultation. You cannot compensate for deficiencies in one domain by possessing extra skills in another domain e.g. a fantastic communicator with very little core knowledge will make a poor clinician, a really good problem solver who cannot communicate effectively with his/her patients will also make a poor clinician. You will need to use different learning techniques to acquire these skills.

Finally, it is important to appreciate that the appropriately-conducted consultation has an intrinsic therapeutic function which can be difficult for students to appreciate until patients tell them how much better they feel after having spoken to the doctor.

References

[1] *Working Party of the Royal College of General Practitioners.* 1972.

[2] Smith S. *Making Medical Minutes Matter. Medical Consultation Skills.* 2010. Litho Press.

In: Learning Clinical Skills
Editors: Bridget Maher and Pat Henn

ISBN: 978-1-62100-409-7

Chapter II

Persistent Cough

Marcus P. Kennedy

Clinical Case

A sixty year old male presented to the clinic with a persistent cough for eight weeks. For the past few years, especially when he gets "chest colds", he suffers from a morning cough productive of sputum. However, the character of the cough had changed. He stated that his cough was now present throughout the day and sometimes disturbs both his and his wife's sleep. He described his cough as an irritating cough and non-productive of sputum during the day, apart from some clear sputum in the morning (Table 1).

He stated that irritants such as aerosolised deodorants, dust and smoke aggravated his cough. He had tried a number of cough suppressants and they did not work. He admitted to some shortness of breath on exertion, especially when walking up a steep hill. He also complained of an occasional wheeze. The wheeze occurred with "chest colds" but also with exertion and was sometimes present in the morning. The patient did not complain of haemoptysis, chest pain, nasal discharge or post-nasal drip. There was no history of dyspepsia. His appetite and weight were stable and he had no fever.

Past Medical History: hyperlipidaemia, hypertension.
Medications: amlodipine and atorvastatin.

The patient's family history was non-significant. He had a 35- 1 pack year smoking history and was a current smoker (Table 2). He drank six units of alcohol at the weekend and denied any illicit drug use. He was married with three children, all well. He worked as a bank manager and denied any occupational or recreational exposure to agents associated with lung disease. He had one pet Labrador at home (kept outdoors).

Table 1. Common respiratory and extrapulmonary causes of acute and chronic cough

	Character of Cough	Associated Symptoms
Respiratory Causes of Cough		
Acute		
Post infectious cough		(runny nose, sore throat, fever) Shortness of breath Wheeze
Asthma	Worse in the night and morning and with exertion. Allergen and irritant exposure	Shortness of breath Wheeze
Bronchitis	Productive	Shortness of breath Wheeze
Pneumonia	Productive	Shortness of breath Fever Pleuritic chest pain
Pulmonary Embolism		Shortness of breath Pleuritic chest Pain
Pneumothorax		Shortness of breath Pleuritic chest pain
Chronic COPD	Worse in the night and morning and with exertion Smoker	Shortness of breath Wheeze
Bronchiectasis	Productive	Shortness of breath Wheeze
Fibrotic Lung Disease	Nonproductive	Shortness of breath
Lung Cancer	Non-productive Change in character	See Table 2
Asthma	Worse in the night and morning and with exertion. Allergen and irritant exposure	Shortness of breath Wheeze
Extrapulmonary Causes of Cough		
Rhinitis Rhinosinusitis	Productive Allergen and irritant exposure.	Nasal discharge, postnasal drip Recent viral prodrome
Gastro-oesophageal Reflux Disease	Often associated with eating	Dyspepsia
Drug-Induced	Associated with commencing drug such as ACE inhibitor	

Table 2. Symptoms and Signs in a smoker which can be associated with lung cancer and warrant further investigation [1]

Symptoms	Signs
• Haemoptysis • New onset of unexplained or persistent cough ≥3 weeks • Alteration in character/severity of cough • Unexplained chest pain or dyspnoea • Unexplained weight loss/cachexia • Unexplained bone pain/neurological symptoms • Hoarseness	• Clubbing • Lymphadenopathy • Focal chest signs • Hepatomegaly • Horner's Syndrome • Asymptomatic hand weakness • Dermatomyositis

Clinical Examination

The patient was positioned at 45 degrees and his chest and abdomen were exposed. He was not hoarse (think vocal cord palsy). From the end of the bed, it was noted that he was not in distress. He coughed on a number of occasions during the history and physical examination. His cough did not sound bovine, brassy, barking or loud. There were no respiratory support devices (oxygen, inhalers, non-invasive ventilation (NIV), nebulizer, or incentive spirometers). His respiratory rate was 14 breaths per minute. His chest appeared symmetrical, there were no scars present and there was no asymmetry of chest wall movement. He did not have accessory muscle use with respiration. His expiratory phase was prolonged in comparison to inspiration. His abdomen moved normally with respiration.

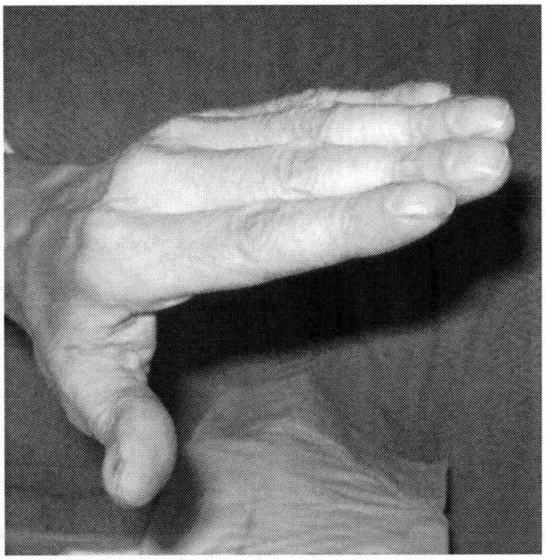

Figure 1. Finger clubbing and tar staining in a 60 yr old male with a cough.

On closer inspection from the patient's right, he had bilateral hand clubbing (Figure 1) and tar staining. His pulse was normal. He had no muscle wasting of his hands (think brachial plexus infiltration by tumour). He had no peripheral or central cyanosis. His pupils and eyelids appeared normal (think Horner's Syndrome). His dentition was normal and no teeth were missing. His oral cavity was normal. On examination of his neck, there was no lymphadenopathy, vessels were not prominent (think Superior Vena Caval obstruction). His trachea was midline, descended by 1 cm, and there was no tracheal tug.

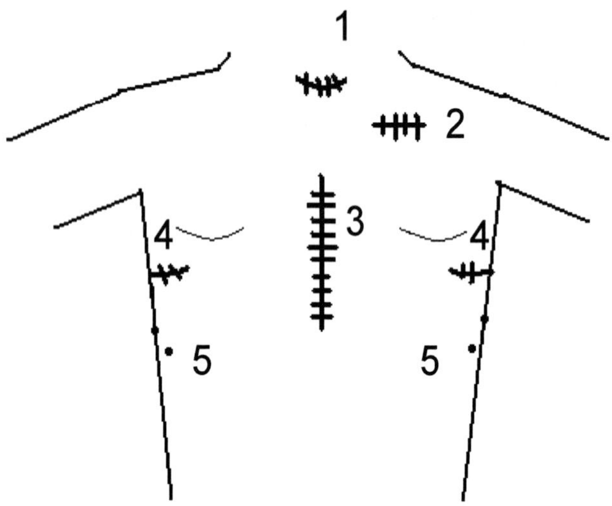

1. Mediastinoscopy scar
2. Left anterior (parasternal) mediastinotomy scar (Chamberlain Procedure)
3. Sternotomy scar
4. Thoracotomy scar
5. Video assisted thorascopy (VATS)/ Pleuroscopy/ Chest drain scars

Figure 2. Surgical Scars and the Respiratory Examination.

Examination of the chest did not identify any surgical scars (Figure 2). On palpation of his chest, chest expansion was normal. His apex beat was not palpable. There was no rib tenderness and vocal fremitus was symmetrical. Percussion of the chest revealed loss of cardiac and liver dullness over his chest.

Auscultation of his chest (Table 4) revealed bilateral but reduced vesicular breath sounds, especially in the upper zones (always describe lung anatomy as zones (left and right upper, middle and lower) rather than lobes unless you are absolutely certain of lobar anatomy as reflected by physical examination. Never use the term "air entry"- you cannot quantify this by stethoscope and patients are often breathing oxygen as inpatients and not air alone. Expiration was prolonged. He had bilateral scattered lower zone crackles (coarse and pan-inspiratory) and bilateral expiratory wheeze. He had no peripheral oedema or cyanosis of his feet. He had bilateral pedal clubbing.

Initial Results: Chest x-ray and an image from his CT thorax are shown in figures 3 and 4. Serum sodium was 129 mmol/l.

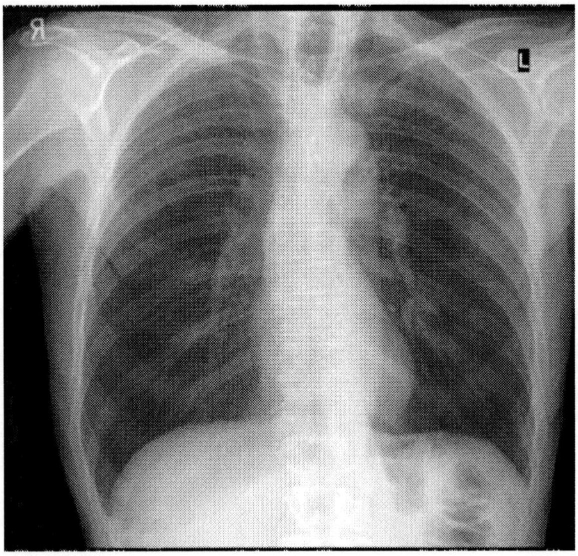

Figure 3. Posterior-anterior chest radiograph displaying hyperinflation and subtle increased shadowing at lower aspect of left hilum in a 60 year old male with cough.

Student Dilemma

The respiratory examination is time consuming if I start at the beginning (end of bed examination) and I work through the hands, face, neck, and chest examination from front, side, and behind. How do I resolve this in practise and in an examination?

What are the most important components of the respiratory examination?

Should I expose the patient's chest for the full examination?

How do I describe chest sounds?

The physical findings I have identified often don't add up to a single disease. How do I summarize findings in this scenario?

Discussion

The majority of respiratory diseases will present with either cough or shortness of breath as a predominant symptom. Disorders of other systems can also present with cough and often there may be characteristics of a patient's cough or associated symptoms and signs which may help in identifying the source (Table 1). The duration of cough is subdivided into two groups - acute (≤8 weeks) and chronic (>8weeks). Symptoms and signs associated with the development of lung cancer in smokers have been identified and should lead to rapid review by a specialist (including chest x-ray) (Table 2).[1] These symptoms include new onset of unexplained or persistent cough ≥3 weeks and a change in the character of the cough.

The examination of the respiratory system is a lengthy process from the initial end of bed inspection, followed by the examination of the chest from the front and behind and the final peripheral examination. It is unusual that an examiner will let you complete the entire examination. Thus, a good start is important, and the place to start is at the end of the bed. A systematic approach for each patient is important and the list presented in Table 3 may be useful (Table 3). I would argue that this is the most important component of the respiratory examination as it will identify whether the patient is acutely unwell and it focuses the rest of your examination. It also creates a good first impression if you perform well here.

Often, after initial inspection, the examiner will ask you to focus in on the chest from in front or behind the patient. You should expose the patient's chest and upper abdomen fully for the examination. Either way, do not forget to inspect, palpate and percuss the flanks- as many important signs such as a thoracotomy scar (Figure 2) or right middle lobe infiltrate may be missed. If the examiner does not direct you, I would advise that you state what you plan to do ("I am going to examine the patient from in front") and proceed. Do not miss a shingles rash as a cause of chest pain!

The trachea should be checked for three features – midline location, descent and tug. Know the difference between descent (permanently down) and tug (moves up and down with respiration).

Regarding palpation, remember to warm your hands. Palpate the chest throughout for tenderness. When assessing for chest expansion, you need to grip the ribcage tight without causing discomfort to prevent the chest expanding and sliding along under your palms without your hands moving. Assessing chest expansion, vocal fremitus and percussion can be practised on a person with a normal respiratory examination. Percussion should be frequently practised. To attain a good percussion note, hyperextend the finger being percussed. The "percussing" finger should not be left on the finger being percussed after the second percussion tap.

Table 3. The end of bed Respiratory Examination.
A systematic approach will focus your respiratory examination and gain points in a clinical examination

Observation	Comment
Respiratory Support Devices	Oxygen, inhalers, nebulisers, non-invasive ventilation, chest drain, sputum jar, incentive spirometers, peak flow meter- know what they look like!
Cyanosis	Present or absent
Respiratory rate	Be precise- avoid "about"
Chest appearance	Symmetrical or not, scars
Chest expansion	Both sides expanding?
Length of inspiration and expiration	Patients can vary this- be careful and observe quiet breathing
Accessory muscle use	Present or absent
Supraclavicular, intercostal recession, pursed lip breathing	Obstructive airway disease associated signs.
Abdominal movement	Normal or paradoxical
Confirm chest expansion	Ask patient to take a deep breath to confirm your initial inspection on quiet breathing
Character of cough, stridor	Comment if patient coughs or if you hear stridor

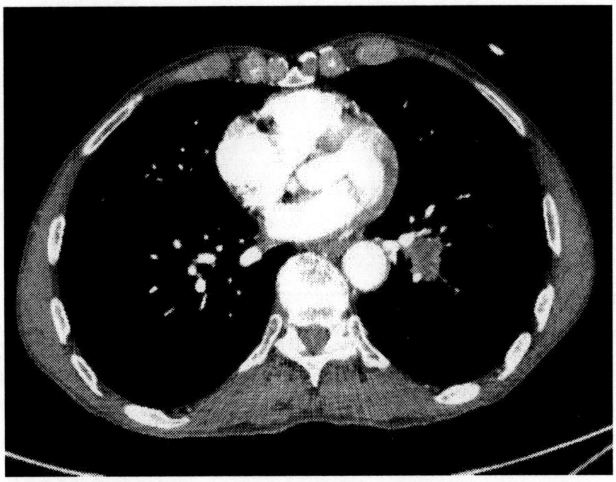

Figure 4. Axial CT thorax with IV contrast image displaying a left hilar mass in a 60 year old male with cough.

Regarding auscultation, there are a number of characteristics of breath sounds which need to be addressed. Having a systematic way of approaching this will again improve your presentation of the respiratory examination and, in practise, help you find more important signs (Table 4). Remember, do not use the term "air entry", the term "breath sounds" is better. Breath sounds should be described anatomically in "zones" rather than "lobes".

Summarising your findings is another important skill to develop during your medical training. It is important to include the pertinent clinical findings and relevant negative findings. It is also important to try and create a cohesive diagnosis from these findings. However, in some respiratory cases, like the patient described here, two diagnoses can be present. Practise by summarising the patient above before reading on.

Table 4. Breath Sounds

Breath Sounds		
Presence	Present	Absent
Intensity	Normal	Reduced
Quality	Normal (vesicular)	Bronchial
Added Sounds		
Crackles	Coarse (usually present early in inspiration or paninspiratory) • Infection • Bronchitis • Pulmonary Oedema	Fine (usually louder in late inspiration) • Pulmonary Fibrosis
Wheeze	Monophonic • (Rare) • Foreign body • Tumour	Polyphonic (Airway disease -asthma, COPD- usually louder in expiration)
Pleural Rub	End-inspiratory crunch	

This patient was a sixty year old current smoker who presented with a new persistent cough. He had signs of chronic obstructive pulmonary disease (COPD) including prolonged expiration, tracheal descent, hyper-resonance to percussion and reduced breath sounds with crackles and wheeze. He also had clubbing which is not consistent with COPD (Figure 1). There are a number of different respiratory diseases that may be associated with clubbing, however clubbing in a smoker should lead to a search for lung cancer (Table 2). This patient's chest X-Ray and CT scan were suspicious for lung cancer (Figures 2, 3) and diagnosis was confirmed by bronchoscopy plus endobronchial ultrasound guided transbronchial needle aspiration (EBUS-TBNA). This patient had no evidence of nodal or metastatic disease, was staged as T2aN0M0, stage 2A and proceeded to surgical resection.[2] Unfortunately, the majority of patients with lung cancer do not present early in the disease and thus there is a drive towards earlier diagnosis and screening.[2]

Lab-spot

Focus on- Electrolyte Abnormalities and Lung Cancer

1. *Sodium-* lung cancer is a frequent cause of the Syndrome of Inappropriate Anti-Diuretic Hormone secretion (SIADH). This can cause hyponatraemia and increased urinary excretion of sodium and can lead to confusion and seizures. On occasion, lung cancer can be associated with hypernatremia and other manifestations of Cushing's syndrome (hypertension, oedema and hypokalaemia). Both these disorders are usually associated with small cell lung cancer.
2. *Calcium-* hypercalcaemia can be associated with tumour secretion of a parathyroid hormone-related protein (PTHrP) and with skeletal metastases. This occurs more commonly with NSCLC (squamous cell).
3. *Potassium-* hypokalaemia can occur with Cushing's Syndrome as described above.
4. *Glucose-* hypoglycaemia can occur due to insulin secretion from lung cancer.
5. Lactic acidosis can rarely be associated with lung cancer.

Pitfalls

- Don't describe physical findings by lobar anatomy, not unless you are sure of your anatomy!
- Don't use the term "air entry". Use the term "breath sounds" instead.
- Know the difference between an NIV machine and a nebuliser and all the respiratory support devices.
- Position the patient correctly and remember to warm your hands.
- Don't miss thoracic scars.

Pearls

- Don't jump in and start inspecting the hands. Have a systematic approach to the end of bed respiratory examination (Table 3).
- Have a systematic approach to describing breath sounds (Table 4).
- Know the different added breath sounds and how to describe them.
- Practise measuring chest expansion and percussion on normal volunteers.
- Always examine the sides of the chest regardless of whether you are asked to inspect the chest from in front or behind.
- In a patient who smokes, be aware of the symptoms and signs associated with lung cancer (warrant further investigation).
- Don't forget to obtain a thorough smoking history; a large proportion of patients attending the respiratory service have smoking related lung disease.

Table 5. Respiratory Causes of Clubbing

Common	Rare
Lung Cancer	Lung Abscess
Bronchiectasis	Empyema
Idiopathic Pulmonary Fibrosis	Asbestosis
	Mesothelioma

Tips for the OSCE

- Remember to look for respiratory support devices.
- Be systematic in your approach to the respiratory exam.
- Practise summarising your physical findings with a summary diagnosis.

Student Check-List

- Describe the characteristics of different types of cough. What is the differential diagnosis of cough?
- What are the steps to the respiratory end of bed examination?
- How do I describe breath sounds?

It Happened to me

Larry was a 35-year-old Chemistry Professor who presented with recurrent pulmonary infection and shortness of breath. He had two prior chest x-rays in two different institutions which displayed some bronchial thickening in his lower lobes consistent with bronchiectasis.

He and his partner were having difficulty conceiving children and a semen analysis confirmed immotile sperm. Thus a differential diagnosis of Primary Ciliary Dyskinesia and non-classic Cystic Fibrosis arose.

On physical examination, no apex beat was palpable on his left side. He had dullness to percussion anteriorally over his left lower ribcage. On auscultation, his heart sounds appeared louder on the right hand side, and a pulsation consistent with an apex beat was palpable on the right. I rechecked the two x-rays; his heart, liver and stomach were definitely on the normal side on x-ray. Perplexed, I grabbed an ultrasound machine and confirmed dextrocardia. Repeat chest x-ray confirmed situs inversus totalis. Thus the patient had a diagnosis of Kartagener's syndrome, a subset of Primary Ciliary Dyskinesia. Both prior x-rays had been labelled incorrectly (the left side of the patient labelled as "right" on the x-ray).

Moral: Trust the physical findings you elicit. Even if previous data suggest different physical findings, or if someone states that the patient has a physical finding that does not match what you find, trust your own examination skills. If you have performed the examination correctly, your findings are correct. The information you have been given could be incorrect, or the physical findings may have changed (e.g. pneumothorax or pleural effusion on top of prior airway disease).

> *I am at the moment deaf in the ears, hoarse in the throat, red in the nose, green in the gills, damp in the eyes, twitchy in the joints and fractious in temper from a most intolerable and oppressive cold.*
>
> Charles Dickens

References

[1] *National Cancer Control Program.* http://www e.ie/eng/servicesFind_a_ Service/ National_Cancer_Control_Programme/Health_Professional_Information/Lung_Guidelines.pdf.

[2] Groome, PA, Bolejack, V, Crowley, JJ, et al. The IASLC Lung Cancer Staging Project: validation of the proposals for revision of the T, N, and M descriptors and consequent stage groupings in the forthcoming (seventh) edition of the TNM classification of malignant tumours. *J Thorac Oncol* 2007; 2:694-705.

In: Learning Clinical Skills
Editors: Bridget Maher and Pat Henn
ISBN: 978-1-62100-409-7

Chapter III

Murmurs, Heart Sounds and More

David Kerins and Carl Vaughan

Clinical Case

A 72 year old male is referred for further evaluation of progressive symptoms of shortness of breath (currently present on climbing one flight of stairs), substernal chest discomfort on exertion and one episode of loss of consciousness. About a year ago, he first noticed shortness of breath on walking his dog but for the past three weeks, has not been able to walk uphill because of shortness of breath. He describes substernal discomfort ("not a pain"), that occurs with exertion and also with stress. He noted a fainting spell that occurred during a strenuous walk on a warm day.

Past medical history: Long standing type II Diabetes Mellitus and hypertension. His fasting cholesterol was elevated when initially checked at the age of 68 years. He was first told that he had a heart murmur approximately 15 years ago. His medications are metformin, a beta-blocker and an hydroxymethylglutaryl CoA reductase inhibitor (statin).

Social history: he has smoked one pack a day of cigarettes since the age of 16 years of age. He denies the consumption of alcohol.

Family history and review of systems: noncontributory.

Clinical examination: the patient is in no obvious distress. Temperature 38.4 C. Blood pressure 138/88 mm/Hg in both arms. Respiratory rate 16/min. Pulse 80 beats per minute and regular.

Table 1. Student Dilemma

- Is this a systolic or diastolic murmur?
- How do I know that this isn't mitral regurgitation?
- What physical maneuvers can help me determine the nature of the patient's valve disease?
- What are the treatment options for this patient?

Examination of the cardiovascular system revealed normal central venous pressure. The carotid upstrokes were decreased in volume and exhibited a delayed upstroke. Palpation of the precordium revealed a forceful sustained apical impulse that was located at the fifth intercostal space in the mid-clavicular line. There was a grade III/VI, late peaking crescendo-decrescendo murmur that was loudest at the right upper sternal border and radiated to the right carotid artery, but was also audible at the left ventricular apex. The murmur was louder over the right clavicle. The aortic component of the second heart sound was absent. A fourth heart sound was audible. Examination of the respiratory system was unremarkable. Abdomen: unremarkable –no pulsatile masses or bruits.

Initial results: FBC normal, fasting blood glucose 8 mmol/l, LDL 2.6 mmol/l, electrolytes, renal function and urinalysis were normal.

Diagnosis: Aortic stenosis.

Discussion

The patient has a systolic murmur. Potential causes for a systolic murmur that are commonly encountered in clinical practice include aortic stenosis, mitral regurgitation, tricuspid regurgitation and hypertrophic cardiomyopathy. Palpation may offer the initial clues in the differentiation between these lesions. In aortic stenosis, the rate of rise of the lightly palpated carotid pulse will be delayed, and the volume will be decreased. The sensation of the pulse over the carotid arteries may resemble a thrill. The interval between the apical impulse and the carotid impulse will be prolonged (apical-carotid delay) in aortic stenosis. The pulse volume is usually normal in mitral regurgitation and in tricuspid regurgitation. Tricuspid regurgitation can lead to the presence of pedal oedema, tender hepatic congestion and the presence of ascites as well as the presence of a prominent CV wave on examination of the jugular venous pulsations. Patients with hypertrophic cardiomyopathy exhibit a prominent carotid pulse with a spike and dome character. There may be a palpable apical atrial impulse in presystole, as well as a double or even triple apical impulse.

Heart Sounds

Heart sounds are also altered in valvular heart disease. One of the hallmarks of severe aortic stenosis is a decreased, or absent, aortic component of the second heart sound. Additionally, if present, the second heart sound may exhibit paradoxical splitting with a narrowing of splitting on inspiration. Aortic stenosis may be associated with the presence of a fourth heart sound. The presence of a third heart sound is not unusual in the setting of mitral regurgitation, and is not a marker of left ventricular dysfunction or elevation of left ventricular filling pressure, whereas in aortic stenosis, a third heart sound is rare, and is an indicator of left ventricular dysfunction. In mitral regurgitation, the first heart sound may be diminished. In mitral regurgitation, and in the setting of a VSD, the second heart sound will exhibit widened physiological splitting, with an earlier aortic component. The second heart sound is usually normal in hypertrophic cardiomyopathy.

Murmurs

The site and radiation of the murmur may assist in the identification of the underlying lesion. Aortic stenosis typically is loudest at the second right intercostal space and radiates to the right carotid artery and the right clavicle. Mitral regurgitation is maximal at the apex and radiates in a band like fashion to the axilla. Occasionally, however, the murmur of mitral regurgitation may radiate to the right upper sternal border. Tricuspid regurgitation may be loudest at the lower left sternal border and radiates to the right sternal border and the epigastrium. Hypertrophic cardiomyopathy frequently is loudest at the fifth left intercostal space and radiates to the lower left sternal border.

Systolic murmurs are harsh distal to an obstruction and are more musical or blowing in nature proximal to the obstruction. Caution needs to be exercised to avoid mistakenly diagnosing the presence of two distinct clinical entities. In particular, the murmur of aortic stenosis may appear harsh at the base of the heart, but at the apex will appear musical (Gallavardin phenomenon).

Murmurs due to increased aortic flow may occur in the setting of anaemia, fever, hyperthyroidism, as a consequence of increased stroke volume in the setting of significant aortic regurgitation or in the setting of abnormal flow into a dilated aorta.

Patients with a bicuspid aortic valve present with symptomatic aortic stenosis at an earlier age than patients with degenerative aortic stenosis. The initial detection of a patient with bicuspid aortic valve may occur when physical examination reveals the presence of an ejection sound that is followed by an early peaking systolic flow murmur. The ejection sound is an indicator of mobility of the valve leaflets and may be loudest at the apex of the heart, but audible at the base and left sternal border. The bicuspid aortic valve occurs in association with coarctation of the aorta, patent ductus arteriosus and ventricular septal defects. These have characteristic findings on clinical examination i.e. radio-femoral pulse delay and upper extremity hypertension, a "machinery" murmur, and a systolic murmur over the lower sternal border, respectively. A large VSD may also have an associated diastolic flow murmur across the mitral valve.

In contrast to aortic stenosis, the classical murmur of mitral regurgitation is a pansystolic (holosystolic) murmur of steady intensity, whose onset occurs with the first heart sound and ends with, of after, the second heart sound.

Maneuvers: Following the performance of "routine" auscultation, the response of the murmur to maneuvers that result in an increase, decrease, or no change in the intensity of the murmur may help to discriminate the aetiology. The simplest of these are maneuvers to *increase venous return,* via inspiration (a decrease in intrathoracic pressure), or abdominal (not hepatic) compression. These will result in an increase in the murmurs of tricuspid regurgitation and pulmonic stenosis. If a pulmonic click of pulmonic stenosis is present, it will typically decrease on inspiration. The murmurs of mitral regurgitation and ventricular septal defect will be increased by *raising systemic vascular resistance (SVR).* This is most easily performed by simultaneously inflating blood pressure cuffs around both arms to a pressure exceeding systolic blood pressure, and listening to the intensity of the murmur 20 seconds later. Changes in *both venous return and SVR* occur in response to changes in posture, e.g. moving from standing to squatting, or in response to passive leg raising. When venous return and systemic vascular resistance are both decreased e.g. by changing from squatting to standing, the murmur of hypertrophic cardiomyopathy will be increased, and the murmur (and click) of mitral valve prolapse will begin earlier in systole. In contrast, *a decrease in venous return and an increase in SVR* occur during the strain phase of a Valsalva maneuver. This technique, which was first described by Valsalva as a technique of clearing pus from the middle ear, can be performed by having the patient strain against a closed glottis, by bearing down as if having a bowel motion or by attempting to blow air from a firmly closed mouth against the *patient's* finger. This will decrease the murmur of aortic stenosis and increase the murmur of hypertrophic cardiomyopathy.

Perhaps the most serendipitous maneuver is when the patient has premature ventricular complexes (PVCs) during the examination. The intensity of the murmur in the two beats that follow a PVC are compared, the first beat being the post-PVC beat, and the second being the "control". In patients with aortic stenosis or hypertrophic cardiomyopathy, the murmur will increase in intensity for the post PVC beat, but will be unchanged in mitral regurgitation.

ECG from a patient with severe aortic stenosis - shows left ventricular hypertrophy, a left atrial abnormality and left axis deviation.

Table 2. History-taking – Aortic stenosis

- History of a heart murmur
- Symptoms of syncope, angina or dyspnoea
- Bicuspid aortic valve
- Rheumatic heart disease
- Calcific degenerative aortic valve disease

Table 3. Risk factors for calcific aortic stenosis

- Hypertension
- Elevated LDL cholesterol
- Male gender
- Smoking
- Diabetes mellitus
- Coronary artery disease
- Chronic renal disease

Table 4. Traditional areas for cardiac auscultation

- Aortic area: second right interspace, sternal border
- Pulmonic area: second right interspace, sternal border
- Erb's point: third right interspace, sternal border
- Tricuspid area: left interspace, mid sternal border
- Mitral area: immediately medial to the cardiac apex, usually fifth left interspace, mid-clavicular line

Table 5. Timing the cardiac cycle

- Identify the first heart sound
- Palpate the point of maximal impulse
- S1 usually louder at the cardiac apex
- S2 usually louder at the base of the heart
- Palpate the carotid upstroke
- At heart rates less than 90 bpm, diastole will be longer than systole

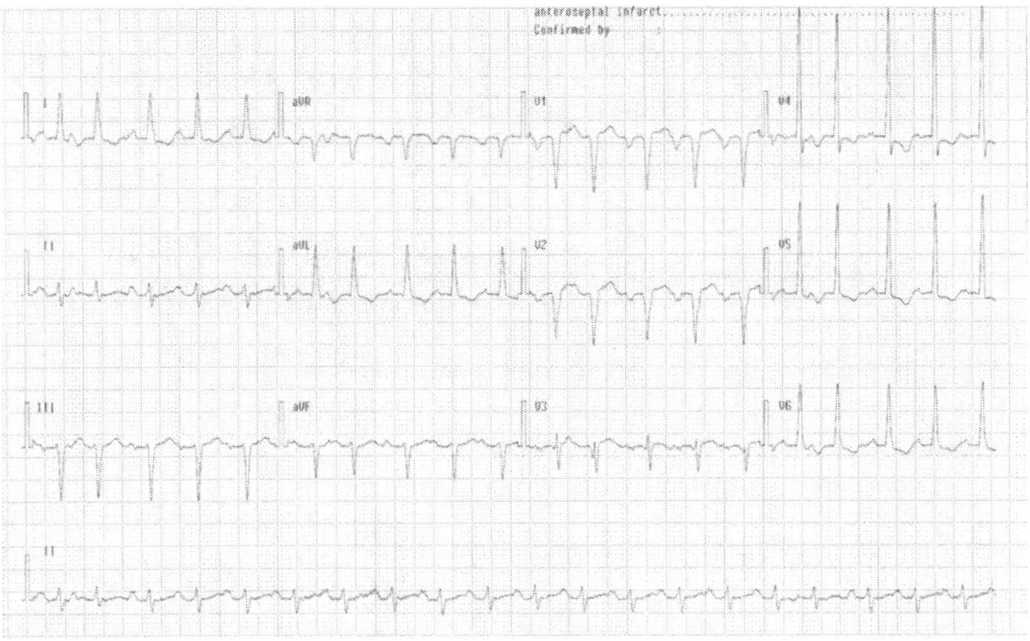

Figure 1. ECG in the setting of aortic stenosis.

Pitfalls

- Always listen in a quiet environment, with a well-maintained stethoscope with well fitting earpieces.
- The murmur of aortic stenosis may be soft, but attention should be focused on the late systolic peaking and its prolonged duration.
- The amplitude and contour of the carotid upstroke are less reliable in the assessment of the severity of aortic stenosis in elderly patients who have co-existing hypertension or a noncompliant vascular tree.
- A patient with typical chest pain and aortic stenosis has symptomatic aortic stenosis and should not undergo exercise treadmill testing.

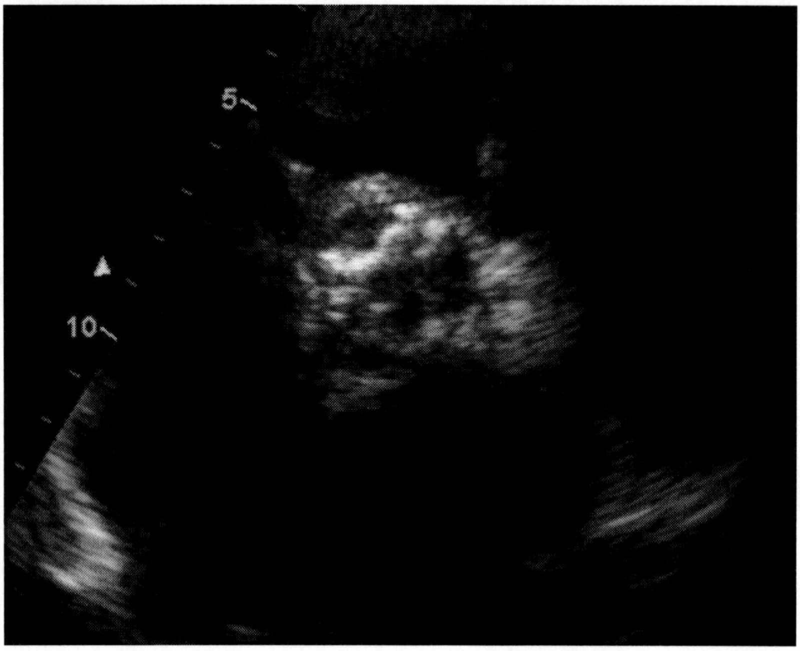

Figure 2. Severe calcific aortic stenosis.

Short axis echocardiographic view of a heavily calcified aortic valve with fusion of the leaflets and decreased valve opening in systole (image courtesy Ms Orla Murray).

Pearls

- When enquiring about the presence or absence of symptoms in a patient with aortic stenosis, always determine the specific level of exertion. Patients may restrict their lifestyle activities to minimise symptoms.
- The traditionally recognized risk factors for atherosclerosis are also recognized as risk factors for the development of aortic stenosis.
- The presence of a normal electrocardiogram makes a diagnosis of significant aortic stenosis unlikely.
- Physical findings that suggest the presence of severe aortic stenosis include a late peaking murmur, diminished carotid pulse upstroke and absence of the aortic component of the second heart sound.
- Bicuspid aortic valve disease is associated with an increased incidence of coarctation of the aorta; if both are present the patient is at increased risk for aortic dissection.
- Listen to one auditory event at a time; focus on the identification of the first heart sound and the second heart sound and characterize events as occurring during systole or during the early or late phases of diastole.
- Clinical assessment is critical in the assessment of patients with aortic stenosis; 50% of patients who present with chest pain survive 5 years, the median survival of

patients who present with syncope is 3 years, but only 2 years in patients who present with congestive heart failure.

- Once patients develop symptomatic aortic stenosis, they should be considered for aortic valve replacement.
- In patients with severe left ventricular failure, and a reduction in cardiac output, the murmur of aortic stenosis may disappear and become "silent"; however, the carotid pulse will exhibit a delayed upstroke.

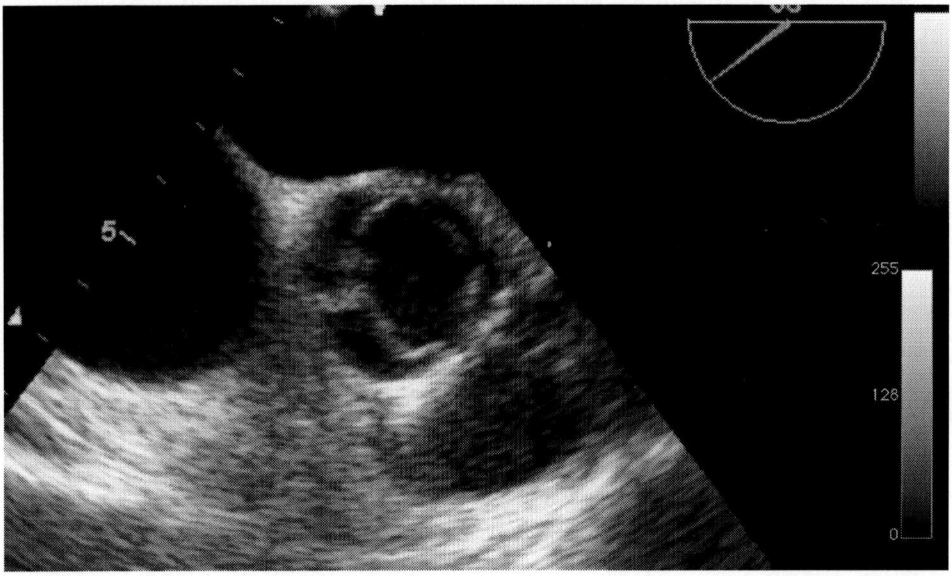

Figure 3. Bicuspid aortic valve.
Transesophageal echocardiogram from a patient with a bicuspid aortic valve. The valve exhibits two leaflets in systole, with the presence of a raphe at the 9 o'clock position.

Table 6. Lab-Spot

Focus on - *Echocardiography*

- Echocardiography will reveal the anatomy of the valve leaflets
  - Calcific degenerative vs bicuspid vs rheumatic
- Allows an assessment of the haemodynamics
- Severe aortic stenosis
  - Peak jet velocity > 4 m/sec
  - Mean gradient > 50 mm Hg
  - Aortic valve area < 1.0 cm^2
- Allows an assessment of the ventricular response to aortic stenosis
  - Left ventricular hypertrophy
  - Left ventricular diastolic dysfunction
  - Left ventricular systolic dysfunction

Tips for the OSCE

- Be courteous and polite. Always explain clearly to the patient what you are going to do and what you want him to do.
- Be confident in your identification of systole and diastole.
- Know the cardiac cycle and the timing of valve closing and chamber filling. You should know when valves are closed and when they are open.
- Be very familiar with the heart sounds and murmurs that occur in systole, in early diastole and in late diastole.

Student Check-List

- Where do you listen for the various heart valves?
- How do you distinguish systole from diastole?
- How do you distinguish aortic stenosis from mitral regurgitation?

It Happened to me

A 45 year-old man with a background of polycythaemia rubra vera presented to the Emergency Department with severe retrosternal pain that had begun one hour prior to presentation. His electrocardiogram demonstrated infero-lateral ST elevation consistent with acute cardiac injury. He was given aspirin, clopidogrel and morphine and was taken to the cardiac catheterization laboratory for primary percutaneous revascularisation. The right coronary was dominant and occluded in the mid vessel. Intravenous heparin and abciximab were administered and thrombus aspiration performed. TIMI-3 flow in the vessel was established and the culprit lesion treated with a drug eluting stent. The patient recovered well and returned to the coronary care unit.

The patient experienced sudden arterial oxygen desaturation on hospital day two. I experienced a new holosystolic blowing murmur at the apex radiating to the axilla. Urgent chest X-ray showed pulmonary oedema. A clinical diagnosis of acute mitral valve regurgitation was made. A portable bedside echo confirmed the diagnosis showing a severe jet of central mitral regurgitation with a flail anterior mitral valve leaflet.

The patient was commenced on intravenous sodium nitroprusside and given IV frusemide and oxygen. He stabilized and had a trans-oesophageal echocardiogram performed and was sent for emergency mitral valve surgery. At surgery, it was noted that he had partial rupture of the postero-medial papillary muscle. The mitral valve was replaced with a mechanical prosthesis and the patient made an excellent recovery.

Clinical examination of patients in the coronary care unit after myocardial infarction is designed to detect new onset heart failure and the mechanical complications of infarction. A new systolic murmur should prompt rapid assessment for either rupture of the papillary apparatus or ventricular septal rupture. These entities can easily be differentiated by bedside echocardiography. Post infarction pericarditis can also manifest with a new “murmur” which is truly a pericardial friction rub. Rupture of the postero-medial papillary muscle is more common than involvement of the antero-lateral muscle as the antero-lateral papillary muscle has a dual blood supply from the left anterior descending and left circumflex arteries. In contrast, the postero-medial muscle has a single blood supply from the posterior descending coronary artery.

Moral: always consider the possibility of the mechanical complications of acute myocardial infarction, including papillary muscle rupture. Emergency surgery can be life saving. Keep valvular heart disease always on your radar!

“We only recognize what we look for, we recognize only what we know”

Merrill C. Sosman

In: Learning Clinical Skills
Editors: Bridget Maher and Pat Henn

ISBN: 978-1-62100-409-7

Chapter IV

Diarrhoea: A Common Symptom

Eamonn M. Quigley

Clinical Cases

A 19 year old student presents with a three month history of worsening diarrhoea. Diarrhoea begins first thing in the morning, is also precipitated by meals and has occurred at night on several occasions necessitating night-time trips to the bathroom. In total, he now passes 5-10 bowel movements over a 24 hour period. Stools are very loose and usually watery and, in the past two weeks, have contained a significant amount of blood which has greatly alarmed him. Initially, he thought that he had a bad case of "food poisoning" but now he is worried that he may have "something more serious".

Immediately before each episode of diarrhoea, he develops a crampy pain in the lower abdomen and then knows that he has to get to the bathroom very quickly; otherwise he fears that he may have "an accident". He thinks that he has lost some weight over the past three months but as he is not in the habit of weighing himself, is unsure of the exact amount. His parents have noticed weight loss and are very worried about him.

Past medical history: fractured humerus at the age of 11.

Social history: commenced smoking at the age of 16 and smoked approximately 10 cigarettes/day but stopped 6 months ago. He "has a few beers at the weekend". He is currently a first year engineering student at university and has missed approximately 25% of his classes because of episodes of diarrhoea, his fear of sudden onset of diarrhoea and urgency in the middle of a class, and feeling very tired.

Family history: his mother has been seen by a gastroenterologist for irritable bowel syndrome. First cousin has Crohn's disease.

Medications: given a 10-day course of ciprofloxacin by his family doctor at onset of symptoms; since then has taken over-the-counter loperamide on an occasional basis which has resulted in some reduction in diarrhoea.

Clinical examination: vital signs normal, afebrile, rather thin but not cachectic. Conjunctiva look pale; examination of head and neck otherwise normal. No skin rash; no arthropathy, 1+ ankle oedema, no sacral oedema, no lymphadenopathy. Cardiovascular and respiratory examination normal.

Abdominal examination: abdomen not distended, slight tenderness on deep palpation in both lower quadrants. No masses, no organomegaly. Rectal examination: no masses but blood on the glove.

Diagnosis: ulcerative colitis.

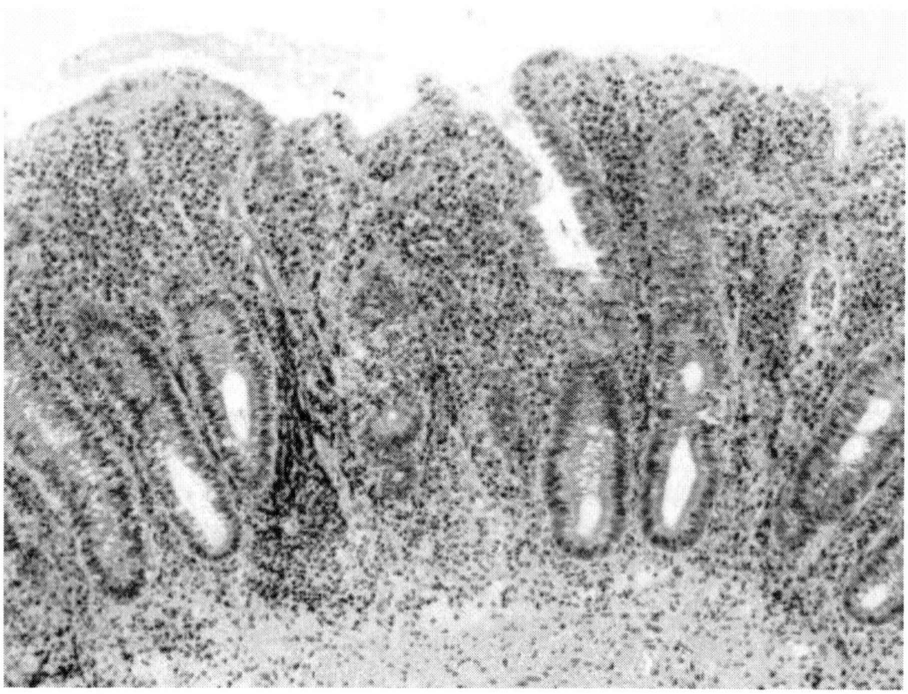

Figure 1. Ulcerative Colitis - Histological features. Marked mucosal lymphocytic infiltration and crypt distortion.

Case 2

A 23-year old female presents with a 13 month history of diarrhoea and abdominal pain. Her symptoms are quite episodic in that she will experience "good" and "bad" weeks. On a "good" week she will be pain free and have a formed bowel movement either once a day or every other day. On a "bad" week she will have bouts of left lower quadrant pain which make her feel as if she needs to have a bowel movement and, as a consequence, she has 3-4 bowel movements per day. Having a bowel movement eases the pain considerably, though she sometimes feels as if the bowel action had been incomplete and "there is still something there". These episodes are most likely to occur within 30 minutes of meals. Though she describes her bowel habit as "diarrhoea", on direct questioning it becomes clear that stools are, for the most part, formed or semi-formed, and are accompanied by some mucus but no blood. In the "bad" weeks, she also describes a sensation of bloating that progresses through the day and is accompanied by visible abdominal distension to a degree that she looks "6 months pregnant" and feels very embarrassed by the end of the day. There has been no weight loss. Periods are regular but she has noticed that she tends to be somewhat constipated towards mid cycle and then has more frequent bowel movements once menstruation commences.

Past History: tonsillectomy age 7. Tended to be constipated as a child.

Table 1. Student Dilemma

- What features of the clinical history help to differentiate between various causes of diarrhoea?
- In a patient with suspected or known inflammatory bowel disease, what specific items need to be addressed in the history and what must be paid special attention to on the physical examination?
- How do I make a diagnosis of irritable bowel syndrome?
- What are "alarm" symptoms and signs?

Table 2. Assessment of the Patient with Diarrhoea –Pearls

- Always aim to understand exactly what the patient means by the term "diarrhoea"; is it really diarrhoea or just frequent formed stools, as is frequently the case in IBS?
- Clearly define the relationship between diarrhoea and pain or discomfort (if present).
- Does the history suggest lower GI or a more small bowel/proximal colon origin? For example, patients with proctitis commonly complain of tenesmus whereas diarrhoea of more proximal origin tends to be large volume.
- Always ask if the patient has incontinence; because of embarrassment, some patients may not volunteer this symptom but instead will state that they have diarrhoea.
- Define the time course, mode of onset and the circumstances in which diarrhoea occurred. Does the history suggest an infectious origin, food poisoning, traveller's diarrhoea?
- Are there symptoms and signs suggestive of systemic upset: fever, anaemia, weight loss, oedema?
- Are there symptoms and/or signs suggestive of a malabsorption syndrome: steatorrhoea, evidence of vitamin deficiency, oedema, weight loss?
- In the family history, always ask specifically about coeliac disease, inflammatory bowel disease (both ulcerative colitis and Crohn's disease) and irritable bowel syndrome.
- Always get a full list of medications; not just prescribed, but also over-the counter and alternative medicines.

Table 3. The Assessment of the Patient with Diarrhoea-Pitfalls

- Not taking an adequate history and simply relying on blood tests, imaging and endoscopy to provide the answers; this is not only wasteful but potentially unethical.
- Failing to appreciate that the patient is having frequent normal stools and not true diarrhoea may lead to the inappropriate prescription of an anti-diarrhoeal medication and exacerbation of the symptoms.
- Failing to recognize that the problem is incontinence and not diarrhoea may lead to a host of unnecessary investigations of no value to the patient.
- Not recognizing symptoms and signs suggestive of inflammatory bowel disease such as ulcerative colitis: weight loss, blood in the stool, anaemia, oedema. Prescribing anti-diarrhoeals in a case of severe ulcerative colitis can precipitate toxic megacolon.
- Missing important clues in the family history.
- Misinterpreting the precipitation of diarrhoea by meals as implying food allergy or intolerance; food allergy and intolerance can cause diarrhoea but virtually all causes of diarrhoea are made worse by eating through the impact of the gastro-colonic response.
- Not thinking of coeliac disease, especially, in a high prevalence population where a simple and highly reliable blood test (tissue transglutaminase) can provide the answer!

Social history: non smoker. Drinks very little alcohol. Works as a secretary in a construction company; considerable stress of late due to the impact of the recession on the construction industry and has had to change her work practice on several occasions over the past year. Constant fear that she may lose her job. *Family history*: two sisters have irritable bowel syndrome.

Medications: has tried herbal products (not sure of name or contents) with no relief.

Clinical examination: vital signs normal, afebrile, looks well. No conjunctival pallor; examination of head and neck normal. No skin rash; no arthropathy, no oedema, no lymphadenopathy. Cardiovascular and respiratory examination normal. Abdominal examination: abdomen not distended. Tender, palpable bowel loop in left lower quadrant. No masses, no organomegaly. Rectal examination: normal but uncomfortable for the patient.

Diagnosis: Irritable Bowel Syndrome (IBS).

Discussion

These two cases, both involving young adults presenting with diarrhoea, illustrate the similarities and differences in symptomatology and physical signs between two common and important causes of gastrointestinal symptoms in this population. Diarrhoea is a symptom that may be readily misinterpreted and several questions need to be addressed by the clinician faced with a patient presenting with this symptom (Table 2). Otherwise, one is likely to fall into one of the pitfalls outlined in Table 3.

Let us now look at the specific features that point to the underlying diagnosis in each of the two cases:

Case 1: Ulcerative Colitis

1. *Clinical History*
    - Young adult
    - Chronic diarrhoea but not much pain
    - Frequent, large volume stools
    - Nocturnal diarrhoea and a lot of diarrhoea in the morning
    - Blood in the stools and not just on the paper
    - Weight loss
    - Fatigue
    - Recently stopped smoking
    - Family history of IBD

2. *Clinical examination*
    - Weight loss
    - Anaemia
    - Oedema (suggests significant protein loss from the inflamed intestine)
    - Abdominal tenderness
    - Blood on the glove on rectal examination

Case 2: Irritable Bowel Syndrome

3. *Clinical History*
    - Young female
    - Chronic episodic symptoms which also fluctuate with menstrual cycle
    - Link between pain and bowel action; precipitation of symptoms by food
    - Not true diarrhoea, but frequent formed/semi-formed stools
    - No nocturnal symptoms
    - Prominent bloating and distension
    - Sense of incomplete rectal evacuation
    - No weight loss or systemic symptoms
    - Past history of constipation
    - Family history
    - Stress at work

4. *Clinical examination*
    - No anaemia, weight loss, oedema
    - Normal abdominal examination apart from the presence of a palpable tender bowel loop in the left iliac fossa, a typical feature of IBS
    - Sensitivity to rectal examination

Remember:

History is all-important in the assessment of the patient with diarrhoea; a failure to take an adequate and thorough history will lead to inappropriate and unnecessary testing and incorrect management.

Additional clinical features that should always be looked for in a patient with ulcerative colitis include, not only evidence of the consequences of active disease (anaemia, weight loss, oedema), but also clinical features relating to the systemic manifestations of inflammatory bowel disease. These are not very common but should always be enquired about on clinical history and sought on physical examination (Table 4).

In *Case 1,* the diagnosis of ulcerative colitis was delayed because of the assumption that this was an episode of food poisoning. However, food poisoning does not cause diarrhoea lasting for three months and should not lead to the late development of bloody diarrhoea. There were many clues in the history and physical examination to suggest the correct diagnosis but because these were not initially detected, an anti-diarrhoeal was inappropriately used. This patient will require full investigation including endoscopy of the colon.

In *Case 2,* in contrast, there is no suggestion of systemic upset and this, otherwise well, young female, has many of the characteristic features of IBS as detailed above. Furthermore, she exhibits none of the "alarm" features or "red flags" (Table 5) that should alert the doctor to consider other diagnoses.

Table 4. Systemic Manifestations of Inflammatory Bowel Disease

- Eye: iritis (Figure 1), episcleritis
- Skin: erythema nodosum, pyoderma gangrenosum, finger clubbing
- Liver: primary sclerosing cholangitis, cholangiocarcinoma, gallstones (Crohn's disease)
- Joints: peripheral arthropathy, sacro-iliitis, ankylosing spondylitis
- Kidney: amyloidosis, renal calculi and urosepsis (Crohn's disease)
- Peri-anal disease (Crohn's disease)

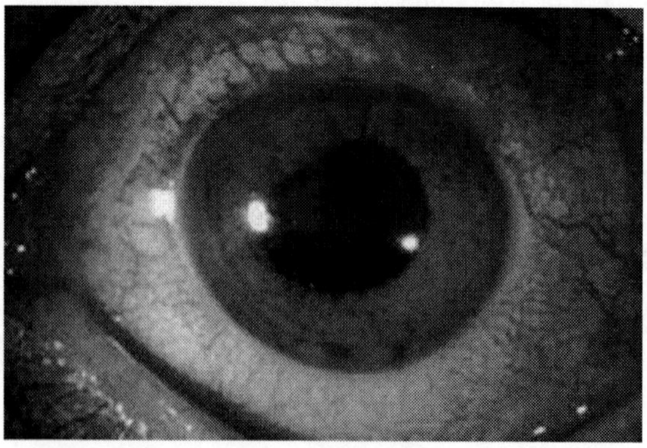

Figure 2. Iritis.

Table 5. 'Alarm Features', 'Red Flags' in IBS

- Onset of symptoms after age 50

- Weight loss
- Fever
- Blood in the stool
- Anaemia
- Oedema

Furthermore, a patient with chronic painless diarrhoea should not be considered as having IBS nor should a patient whose sole complaint is chronic abdominal pain. What then are the cardinal features of IBS?

IBS is defined by the presence of abdominal pain or discomfort which is, in some way or other, associated with bowel action (makes the patient feel that they need to go, or pain is relieved or made worse by going) and is often accompanied by bloating and distension.

Symptoms are typically episodic (bad day/good day, bad week/good week) and are characteristically exacerbated by stress, food and the menstrual cycle. In the correct context, e.g. young female patient, in the presence of compatible symptoms and in the absence of "alarm" features, a clinical diagnosis of IBS is, not only possible, but to be recommended. Furthermore, not only is the clinical encounter critical to the approach to IBS, but the doctor-patient relationship and, in particular, the ability of the doctor to listen to the patient and understand their symptoms and their impact, is vital to the management of this very common condition.

Tips for the OSCE

- Listen to the patient; know exactly what they mean by the term diarrhoea
- Elicit all related symptoms
- Pay attention to past medical history, family history and medication history
- Look for anaemia, oedema, evidence of malabsorption, weight loss
- A normal abdominal examination excludes little but certain findings may be helpful
- Think 'big picture'; try to put the various parts of the story together to narrow the differential diagnosis and help guide investigations

Student Check List

- What is diarrhoea?
- What are common causes of diarrhoea in various age-groups?
- What are the clinical features of infectious diarrhoeas, inflammatory bowel disease, coeliac disease, and irritable bowel syndrome?
- What are the complications of IBD that can be detected on clinical examination?

It Happened to me

I was asked to see a 58 year-old lady who had developed very high output watery diarrhoea resulting in dehydration and the need for intravenous fluid replacement following a cholecystectomy. She had been extensively investigated at the hospital where I saw her and no cause had been found. Knowing that having your gall bladder removed can disrupt the bile salt pool and lead to bile salt diarrhoea, I thought that I was very clever and suggested a bile salt chelating agent. In looking through the patient's chart, I had seen a comment in a hand-written note "duodenal biopsy normal" and accepted it as such. The patient deteriorated further and only later, when we actually reviewed the duodenal biopsy and the pathologist's report, did we realize that the patient had severe coeliac disease. Fortunately, she responded to a gluten-free diet and has been well since.

Moral: common things remain common, even in unusual contexts; never trust hearsay or second hand evidence – check it out yourself!

It is much more important to know what sort of a patient has a disease than what sort of a disease a patient has.

Sir William Osler

In: Learning Clinical Skills
Editors: Bridget Maher and Pat Henn

ISBN: 978-1-62100-409-7

Chapter V

Neurological Examination

Patricia M. Fitzgerald

Topic: Right Hemiparesis

Clinical Case 1

A 70 year old right handed man presents with weakness of his right upper and lower limbs and speech difficulty (onset two hours previously). He is unable to speak but seems to understand what is being said. The history is given by his partner. She noticed that when she woke the patient that morning, the patient's face was distorted and he seemed to have difficulty moving his right limbs. He has not spoken any normal words since onset.

Past medical history: Diabetes Type 2, elevated cholesterol and hypertension (all diagnosed five years ago). His medications are gliclazide, enalapril, and atorvastatin. Social history: smoker, 10 to 20 cigarettes daily for the past 50 years. No alcohol or illicit drug use. There is a family history of ischaemic heart disease. Review of systems non-contributory.

Clinical examination: the patient is distressed. Temperature 38.4C. Blood pressure 160/100 mm/Hg. Respiratory rate 18/min. Pulse 90 bpm - irregularly irregular. Cardiovascular examination: diminished pedal pulses and a left carotid bruit present. Neurological examination: aphasia and right hemiparesis. Right upper limb power 2/5, right lower limb power 4/5. Hemisensory loss and right hemianopia are also evident. He has brisk reflexes on the right with an upgoing plantar response. Examination of the respiratory and gastrointestinal systems is normal.

Clinical Case 2

A 65 year old right handed woman falls to the right while doing her grocery shopping. She calls for help. An observer tries to sit her up but she is unable to move her right limbs. Her face is distorted and her speech in intelligible but dysarthric.

Past medical history: Poorly controlled hypertension for the past 10 years (currently treated with losartan). Social history: non smoker. No alcohol or illicit drug use. Family history is positive for hypertension in three siblings and her mother. Review of systems non-contributory.

Clinical examination: the patient is very upset. Temperature 38.4C. Blood pressure 155/105 mm/Hg. Respiratory rate 18/minute. Pulse rate – 80, regular. Fundoscopy reveals AV nipping but cardiovascular examination is otherwise normal. Neurological examination: dysarthria. Mentation is normal. Right facial weakness is evident with sparing of forehead wrinkling. There are no visual deficits. Weakness is grade 3/5 in the right upper and lower limbs, but sensation is normal. She has brisk reflexes on the right with an upgoing plantar response.

Examination of the respiratory and gastrointestinal systems is normal.

Diagnosis: Right hemiparesis

Discussion

Both patients presented with acute onset right-sided weakness suggestive of vascular disease, but have different associated clinical findings. We have rules to help localize the neurological lesion.

1. Presume that there is only ONE lesion.
2. The lesion is on the side OPPOSITE to the hemiparesis.
3. Where different anatomical pathways are affected, the lesion is where these pathways MEET.

Table 1. Student Dilemma

• Where is the lesion?
• What is the lesion?
• What is common in this age group?
• What caused it?
• What is the treatment?

These patients have right hemiparesis and the lesion can be localized to one of four sites (Figure 1). The situation becomes more complicated when other neurological signs are present. A basic knowledge of motor (Figure 2) and sensory (Figure 3) pathways is vital to localization of the lesion and a basic knowledge of neuroanatomy is essential in neurological history-taking and examination.

Localization of the lesion in Case 1 is not difficult. The patient has hemiparesis, hemisensory loss, hemianopia and aphasia which place the lesion in the left middle cerebral artery territory. Additionally, the patient has multiple risk factors for stroke: atrial fibrillation, diabetes, smoking, hypertension, elevated cholesterol and a positive family history.

Case 2 has a pure motor stroke with a background history of hypertension making a diagnosis of lacunar stroke left internal capsule the most likely diagnosis.

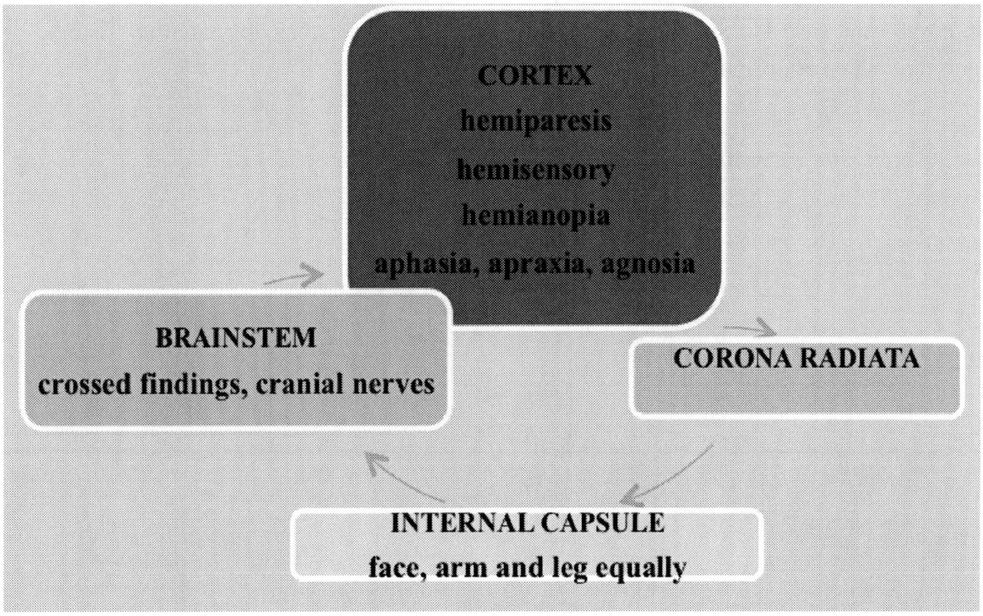

Figure 1. Right Hemiparesis – Localising the Lesion.

Table 2. Neurological History

- Handedness
- Memory
- Cognition
- Headache
- Loss of consciousness or seizure
- Involuntary movements
- Speech difficulty
- Ask about cranial nerves individually
- Weakness/clumsiness of limbs and pattern
- Sensory abnormality of limbs and pattern
- Neck or back pain
- Difficulty walking
- Difficulty with bowel or bladder
- Current state of function

The Neurological History

When assessing a patient with a neurological lesion, the first concern is the NEUROLOGICAL HISTORY. A commonly held view states that you should have a reasonable grasp of the patient's diagnosis after taking the history. Otherwise you are unlikely to find the diagnosis on examination. Important neurological symptoms are listed in Table 2. These should be specifically asked about in the context of the general history. Cardiac symptoms and risk factors for vascular disease, family history, psychiatric history, drug history and sleep abnormalities may be particularly relevant.

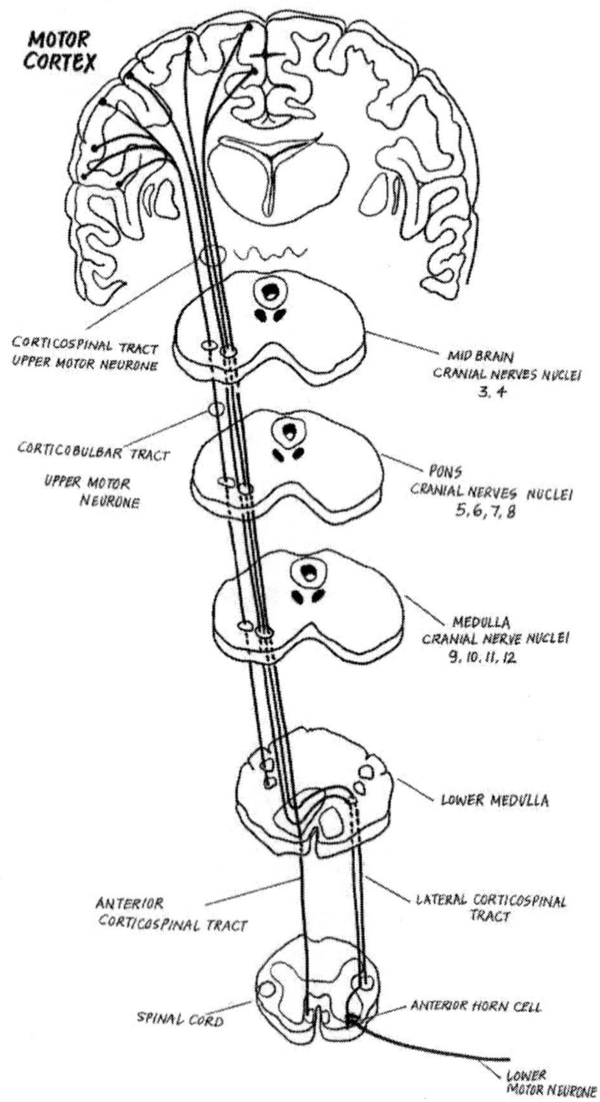

Figure 2. Motor Pathways. Image courtesy of Catherine Mills, School of Medicine, UCC.

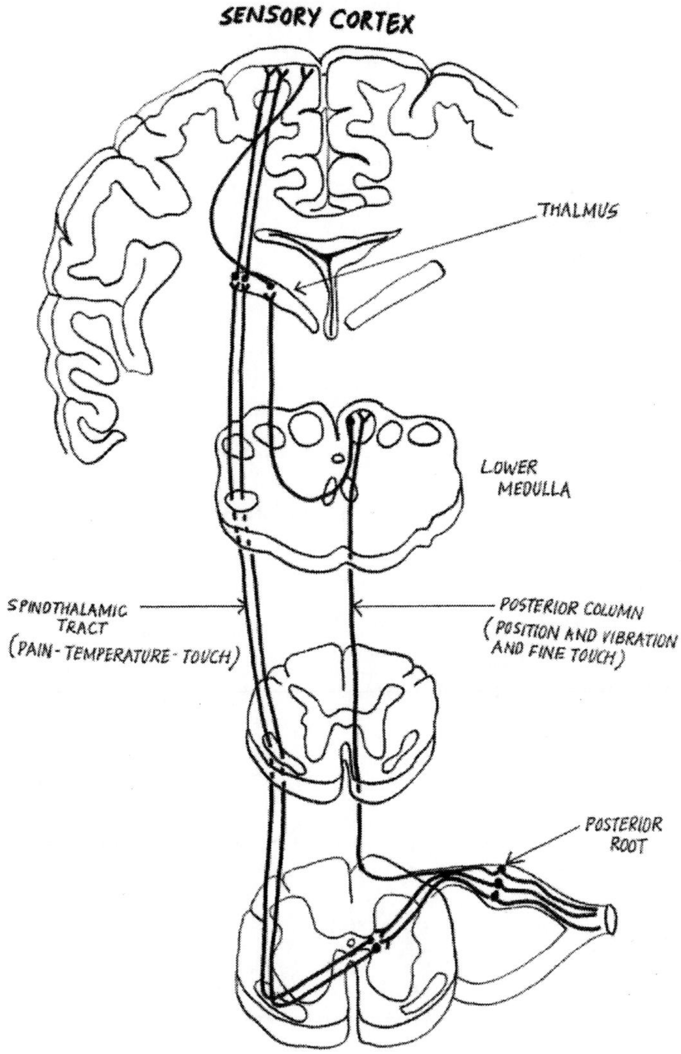

Figure 3. Sensory Pathways. Image courtesy of Catherine Mills, School of Medicine, UCC.

Some symptoms require teasing out in further detail such as headache (Table 3), seizure, and loss of consciousness (Table 4).

The TEMPO of onset is a very helpful guide to the likely etiology of the disease. Both patients had an acute onset of neurological deficit which suggests a vascular basis (in the absence of trauma).

The Neurological Examination

Remember that this is an important record which may change over time. Accuracy in documentation is vital. An examination template ensures that no aspect of the examination is left out. However, examination should also concentrate on areas of abnormality.

Table 3. Headache questions

- Triggers
- Location
- Radiation
- Association
- Pulsation
- Aggravation
- Duration
- Frequency
- Severity
- Relieving factors
- Family history

Table 4. Loss of consciousness questions

- Triggers
- What happened before the event?
- What happened during the event?
- What happened after the event?

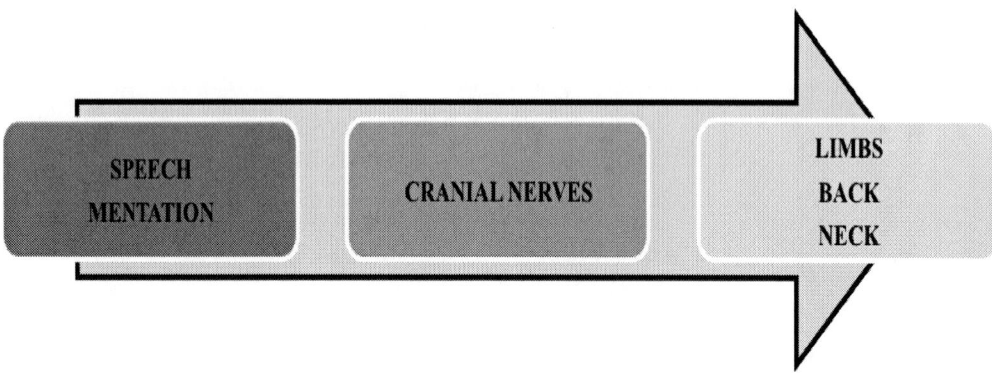

Figure 4. The Neurological Examination.

Table 5. Speech Testing

- Comprehension of speech
- Fluency of output
- Naming
- Repetition
- Reading
- Writing
- Calculation

Speech

Establish that the patient can *understand* speech using a one step command.

Is the patient DEAF or does he have DEMENTIA? If not, then test for speech as in Table 5. Note presence of *dysarthria, dysphonia, dysphasia and dysprosody.*

Testing Cranial Nerves

NERVE	*FUNCTION/S*	*TEST*
1.OLFACTORY	SMELL	SMELL BOTTLES
2. OPTIC	VISION	VISUAL FIELDS - sit at same level as patient - test eyes together and separately - use red and white hat pins VISUAL ACUITY- - Snellen and Jaegar charts FUNDI AFFERENT LIMB LIGHT REFLEX
3.OCULOMOTOR 4. TROCHLEAR 6. ABDUCENS	EYE MOVEMENTS = EOMS PUPILLARY RESPONSE EYELIDS	FOLLOW finger and observe - asymmetry, saccades, pursuit, nystagmus, VOR and convergence COVER TEST PUPIL SIZE and SYMMETRY PUPILLARY RESPONSE - Direct - Consensual and Accommodation - Swinging flashlight test PTOSIS - Parasympathetic - Sympathetic

The patient may need to wear glasses when testing Cranial Nerve 2. Visual fields are described from the patient's perspective.

Figure 5. CRANIAL NERVES: 1, 2, 3, 4, 6 (test 3, 4 and 6 together).

Mentation / Higher Cerebral Function

The MMSE (Mini-Mental Status Examination) is easy to perform [1]. It supplies basic information about speech, but praxis and gnosis may require more detailed testing. The GCS (Glasgow Coma Scale) may be required [2].

NERVE	*FUNCTION/S*	*TEST*
5. TRIGEMINAL A. OPHTHALMIC B. MAXILLARY C. MANDIBULAR MOTOR	SENSATION CORNEAL REFLEX MOTOR	- Temperature and light touch all divisions - Corneal reflex JAW JERK POWER in the Temporalis, Masseter and Pterygoid muscles
7. FACIAL	FACIAL EXPRESSION ACUSIS - STAPEDIUS TASTE ANTERIOR TONGUE TEAR FORMATION	Facial SYMMETRY and corneal reflex Remainder not usually tested unless lower motor seventh lesion present
8. AUDITORY and VESTIBULAR	HEARING BALANCE	RINNE and WEBER performed with 512 Hz tuning fork Turning test Calorics - done in comatose patient
9,10. GLOSSOPHARYNGEAL and VAGUS	SENSORY MOTOR	GAG reflex Say "ah" - uvula and palate symmetry COUGH / SWALLOW
11. ACCESSORY	TRAPEZIUS STERNO-CLEIDOMASTOID	Shrug shoulders Turn head, push forward
12. HYPOGLOSSAL	TONGUE	Observe tongue Observe protruded tongue

Figure 6. Cranial Nerves: 5, 7, 8 – 12. On testing EOMS, ask patient to follow your finger without moving their head. VOR = Vestibulo-ocular reflex.

Examination of the Motor System

Power

- Review root and nerve supply for muscles being tested. [3]
- Test for pronator drift - hold arms extended and supinated at 90 degrees.
- Test for tremor.
- Test *UPPER LIMB* strength bilaterally in: shoulder abduction and adduction, elbow flexion and extension, wrist extension and flexion, finger extension and flexion,

finger adduction and abduction. Thumb adduction (Ulnar nerve) and opposition (Median nerve) should also be checked as should other muscles in determining root lesions.

- Test *LOWER LIMB* strength bilaterally in: hip flexion, extension, abduction, and adduction, knee flexion and extension, ankle dorsiflexion, plantar flexion, inversion, eversion and hallux extension.

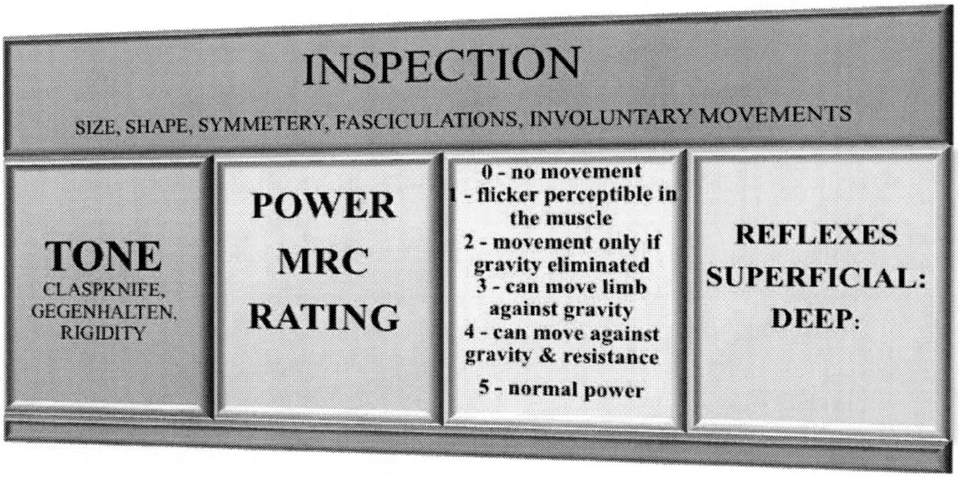

Figure 7. Motor Testing.

WEAKNESS	*ASSOCIATED FINDINGS*
UPPER MOTOR NEURONE	↑ TONE, ↑ REFLEXES, EXTENSOR PLANTARS
LOWER MOTOR NEURONE	↓ TONE, ↓ REFLEXES, WASTING, FASCICULATIONS
MYONEURAL JUNCTION	NORMAL TONE AND REFLEXES, FATIGUABILITY
MUSCLE	PROXIMAL WEAKNESS AND WASTING

Figure 8. Patterns of weakness.

REFLEX	*INNERVATION*
BICEPS	C5,6
SUPINATOR	C5,6
TRICEPS	C7,8
FINGER FLEXOR	C8
KNEE JERK	L3,4
ANKLE JERK	S1,2
PLANTAR RESPONSE	S1

Figure 9. Commonly tested reflexes.

GRADE DESCRIPTION	*MEANING*
0	ABSENT
1+	DIMINISHED
2+	NORMAL
3+	BRISK WITHOUT CLONUS
4+	BRISK WITH CLONUS

Figure 10. Grading of reflexes.

Sensory Nervous System

- A diagram of the body or limbs, illustrating the areas of sensory abnormality is helpful
- Note right versus left, distal versus proximal and dermatomal differences
- *Non-cortical sensory testing:* pain, temperature, light touch, vibration appreciation (128Hz tuning fork)
- *Cortical sensory testing:* position sense, stereognosis, graphaesthesia, tactile localisation

Note: There is no point in cortical sensory testing if the patient cannot feel the non-cortical modalities.

Cerebellar Testing

Midzone functions - head posture, eye movements, titubation, stance and gait.
Lateral zone functions -
D - dysarthria, dysmetria, dysdiadochokinesia
I - intention tremor
R- rebound, reduced tone, reflexes pendular
E - eyes -nystagmus and gaze apraxia

Gait

- Ask the patient to walk, tandem walk, walk on their tip toes and walk on their heels
- Note:
  - shuffling gait or lack of arm swing suggestive of Parkinson's disease
  - hemiparetic gait - stroke
  - ataxic gait - cerebellar disease
  - steppage gait - neuropathy
  - antalgic gait - pain

ROMBERG'S TEST: Test at the same time as gait. Ask the patient to stand with feet together. Then ask the patient to close his/her eyes. Be prepared to catch the patient.

Don't forget to examine the *BACK* and *NECK* - Look for *MENINGISM* and check the *CAROTID* arteries.

Finally, based on your clinical findings, *where do you think the lesion is?*

- Cortex
- Subcortex
- Brainstem
- Cerebellum
- Spinal cord
- Spinal root
- Plexus / Nerve
- Myoneural junction
- Muscle

Pitfalls

- A core understanding of neuroanatomy is *imperative* for studying neurology.
- You should be able to draw a cross section of the midbrain, pons, medulla, spinal cord and the visual pathways from memory.
- Always expose the limbs and trunk fully. Otherwise, you may miss wasting, fasciculations, involuntary movements and asymmetry.
- Don't forget to test tone - hold upper limb and roll. Lift the lower limb.
- Comparison is vitally important and the patient acts as his/her own control. Note differences between right and left but also between distal and proximal.
- The cardiovascular examination is of considerable relevance to the neurological examination as is the autonomic nervous system.
- Don't forget to test gait and Romberg's Test.

Pearls

- If your history taking is inadequate, you will be lost before you start the examination.
- If your examination is inadequate, you will not establish where the lesion is.
- If you do not know where the lesion is, you will not be able to determine what it is.
- Age at onset and tempo of onset are important clues to aetiology of the lesion.
- In speech testing, remember to test whether patients can hear and understand you before testing their ability to speak, name, repeat, read and write.
- Is a MMSE or GCS indicated?

- For visual field testing, have the patient sit at the same level as you and ask him to look at your nose. Test for visual inattention and then test each eye separately by covering each eye in turn.
- When testing Cranial Nerves 3, 4 and 6, don't forget ptosis. Test eye movements slowly so that you do not miss nystagmus.
- Cranial nerves and upper limbs are best tested with the patient seated.
- Lower limbs are best tested with the patient lying down, unless you plan kneeling to test the ankle jerks which could be awkward.
- GAIT testing may reveal subtle neurological signs that are otherwise missed - reduced arm swing in Parkinson's disease, involuntary movements and ataxia.

Tips for the OSCE

- Know what conditions are common and the relevant important physical signs.
- Ask for consent and ask if the patient has pain before starting the examination.
- Give the patient clear instructions.
- Look around the bed for clues (walker, wheelchair).
- Remember that the neurological history points to the important aspects of the examination.
- Have a systematic plan for examination of speech, mentation, cranial nerves, motor systems, sensory systems, reflexes, cerebellum and gait.
- Remember that the purpose of the examination is to determine where the lesion is.
- Practice on your friends and always do a neurological examination on patients even if they have no neurological complaints.

Student Check-List

- Can I take a neurological history?
- How do I do a speech examination?
- Can I perform a MMSE and Glasgow Coma Scale?
- Do I know the anatomical relevance and clinical aspects of CRANIAL NERVE examination?
- Can I do a systematic examination of power in the upper and lower limbs?
- Can I do a sensory examination which includes cortical sensory testing?
- Can I elicit reflexes?

It Happened to me

In patients with hemiparesis and aphasia, apraxia or agnosia with acute onset, a presumption of vascular diagnosis in the middle cerebral territory is generally reasonable, but what if the patient just has right limb weakness, with, for example, left seventh cranial nerve signs and inability to look to the left? Or right hemianaesthesia with vocal cord and soft palate paralysis? These crossed findings with cranial nerve abnormalities point us to the brainstem. For any presentation, we must look for findings which point us to an anatomical level, or away from it.

Pointers to the spinal cord include a sensory level, sphincter disturbance, bilateral findings and hyper-reflexia below the level. Identification of plexus and root lesions requires a basic knowledge of neuroanatomy. Suggestive findings in peripheral neuropathy are bilateral distal weakness and wasting and glove and stocking sensory loss. Myopathy findings include proximal, often painless weakness without sensory loss.

In the fields of observation chance favors only the prepared mind

Pasteur

References

[1] Adapted from Folstein M et al. "Mini-Mental State", a practical method for grading the cognitive state of patients for the clinician. J Psychiatry Res., 1975, Vol 12, 189-198 and Cockrell J et al. Mini-Mental State Examination (MMSE). *Psychopharmacology Bulletin,* 1988, Vol 24, No. 4, 689-692.

[2] Glasgow Coma Scale. Teasdale G, Jennett B. "Assessment of coma and impaired consciousness. A practical scale."*The Lancet* 13;2(7872):81-4, 1974.

[3] *Aids to Examination of the Peripheral Nervous System* 4th edition.2000. Elsevier Saunders.

In: Learning Clinical Skills
Editors: Bridget Maher and Pat Henn

ISBN: 978-1-62100-409-7

Chapter VI

Petechiae and Purpura

Mary R. Cahill

Clinical Case

A fifty year old man attends the clinic because of recent onset bruising on both hands. He has a past history of Immune Thrombocytopenia (ITP) and has been on steroid therapy. On examination, there is obvious skin thinning and classical large steroid purpura on the back of the hands (prolonged steroid therapy). There were small abrasions and ingrained dirt on the finger pads and nail folds. He is right handed and the worsening petechiae and steroid purpura on the right hand are consistent with the physical work of gardening. His ITP has relapsed and his platelet count was $24x10^9/l$. The platelet count is not low enough to cause purely spontaneous skin bleeding as would be expected with counts $<10x10^9/l$. In spontaneous bleeding, laterality is also less likely.

Table 1. Definition of a petechial/purpuric rash

Petechial rash Erythematous (red) spots on the skin due to haemorrhage. Petechiae measure <3mm in diameter. Haemorrhage occurs at skin capillary level.
Purpuric rash (purpura) Erythematous (or sometimes purplish) spots on the skin due to small vessel skin haemorrhage where the size of the spot is >3mm and <1cm.
Ecchymosis (bruising) Red or purple discolouration of the skin measuring > 1cm due to bleeding underneath the skin in larger blood vessels.

Discussion

A patient with thrombocytopenia usually presents for medical assessment because of a "rash". Examine the rash carefully including inspection, palpation and testing for blanching (disappearance on pressure).

Petechiae or Mucosal Bleeding -Taking a History

The patient's medical history should include questions about the onset of the petechiae, the time frame, and any other bleeding (epistaxis, vaginal bleeding, gum bleeding and history of bleeding after dental extractions/surgery/child birth). A history of receiving a blood transfusion may serve as a proxy marker for bleeding and should always be sought. A strong family history brings inherited disorders of coagulation into the differential diagnosis.

In an older patient, a history of infection may point to neutrophil dysfunction and malignant or pre malignant bone marrow disorders such as myelodysplastic syndrome or myeloma should be considered. For this reason, the older patient may benefit from bone marrow sampling (usually not necessary in the younger patient).

It is important to ask about a family history of bleeding. In addition to the usual general questions, attention should focus on the obstetric history of female patients and their relatives. Childbirth is a significant challenge to the haemostatic system. Menstrual history may also be relevant. Answers such as "my great granddad died of a brain haemorrhage" should be probed where possible as a brain "haemorrhage" could just as easily be a brain thrombosis in lay terms. Where probing is unrevealing, the patient's information should be recorded with any supporting information or with a question mark to indicate the history taker's impression that the information may not be definitive

Table 2. Petechial Rash - History Pearls

- Duration of rash
- Sites of rash and any other bleeding
- Heavy periods
- Past history of bleeding
- Family history of bleeding and/or low platelet count
- Drugs – including alternative and complementary therapies.
- History of infection
- Diet (garlic, green tea, any unusual foods) and alcohol
- Other illnesses

As with every patient, the history should include a complete list of regular medications (recorded in generic form) and drugs taken on a *pro re nata* (PRN) basis. For patients with potential bone marrow disorders, it is particularly important to ask about and record any herbal or alternative medicines and vitamin supplements. There are numerous reports of herbal remedies such as Echinacea causing bone marrow side effects. Garlic, alcohol and omega oils can reduce platelet function and exacerbate bleeding in a patient with thrombocytopenia. A meticulous alcohol history recorded in units per week is vital. Table 3 details the differential diagnosis and distinguishing features of a petechial-like rash.

Examination of a Purpuric Rash

Once you have confirmed the petechial nature of the rash, examination of the patient with a petechial rash should include examination of the mouth, teeth and gum line for oral blistering or mucosal petechiae and for areas of periodontal bleeding. Fundoscopy is necessary to assess for ocular haemorrhages (Figure 2) and specialist ophthalmologist review should be requested if any abnormalities are noted. All skin surfaces should be examined. In recumbent hospital inpatients, petechiae may be worse on the buttocks and back, in ambulant patients the shins may be selectively affected (Figure 3).

Examine for other physical signs. In Figure 4, additional clues are found in the presence of skin thinning and larger classical steroid purpura on the back of the hands. These are due to prolonged steroid therapy in a patient on intermittent long-term steroids for Immune Thrombocytopenia (ITP). Notice the small abrasions and ingrained dirt on the finger pads and nail folds of this male patient. He is right handed and the pictures reveal worsening petechiae and steroid purpura on the right hand. This is consistent with the physical work of gardening and indicates that the count is not low enough to cause purely spontaneous skin bleeding as would be expected from counts $<10x10^9/l$. In spontaneous bleeding, laterality is less likely. His ITP has relapsed however, and his platelet count was $24x10^9/l$. Palpate the abdomen for mild splenomegaly (present in only 10-20% of patients with ITP). Any splenic enlargement more than a spleen tip should prompt consideration of other haematological diagnoses and viral infection.

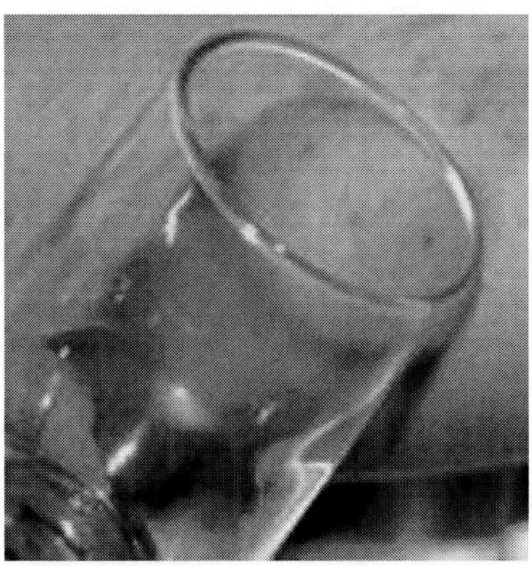

Figure 1. Testing for blanching:when a glass (or finger) is pressed against a petechial rash, the rash remains unchanged and does not blanch. Reproduced by kind permission Meningitis UK. www.meningitisUK.org.

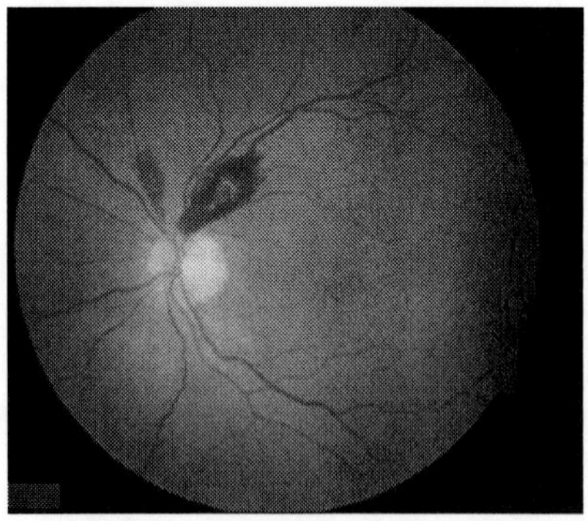

Figure 2. Fundal haemorrhage in a thrombocytopenic patient.

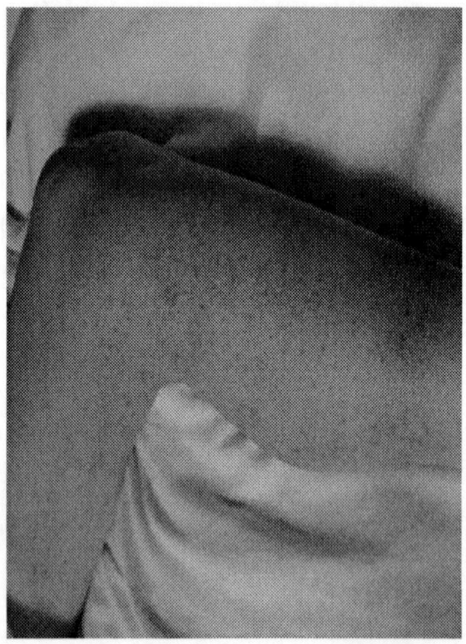

Figure 3. Patient with dependent petechiae undergoing treatment for acute leukaemia with a platelet count $<10x10^9/l$.

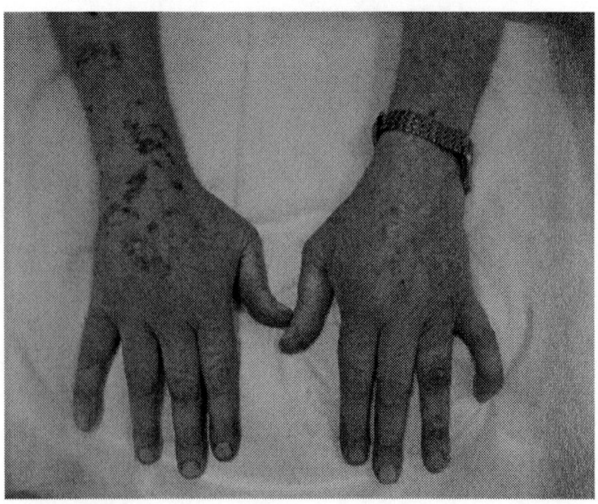

Figure 4. Petechiae, purpura and steroid changes (skin thinning) in a patient with chronic ITP.

Table 3. Differential Diagnosis of Petechial-like rash

Diagnosis	Distinguishing Features	General condition patient	Other remarks
Petechiae due to thrombocytopenia	Flat unblanching red spots <10mm occurring in clusters (figure 2)	Usually well. Short history.	Typically of sudden onset. Traumatic bruise may also be present.
Purpuric rash secondary to meningococcal septicaemia (or other infection)	Flat unblanching rash, clinically undistinguishable from petechiae due to thrombocytopenia but may be more extensive.	Patient typically (but not always) unwell. Non-blanching, changes rapidly with time and may become confluent in the extremities, particularly in children.	This is a critical diagnosis because of the potential for immediate life saving treatment. Possibility of meningococcal septicaemia should always be considered in initial assessment of an apparent petechial rash.
Henoch Schonlein Purpura	Non-blanching rash, typically over buttocks in children and associated with abdominal pain and arthritis.	Unwell – multisystem disorder.	This is an IgA mediated vasculitis. Check urine. History of infection common.
Scurvy	Gums severely affected.	History of vitamin C deficiency or general malnutrition.	Tends to occur with other signs of malnourishment. Consider in malnourished children and the elderly.
Hereditary telangiectasia	Typically occur in the mouth and mucosal surfaces (often only seen on endoscopy).	Well patient. Blanch on pressure and fill from the centre.	Patient may be anaemic. There is a family history. Genetic testing available.
Spider naevae secondary to liver disease	Typically occur over trunk and upper limbs.	Associated with other stigmata of chronic liver disease. Blanch on pressure and fill from the centre.	History usually reveals systemic effects of liver failure and/or cause. Always ask about alcohol consumption.
Campbell de Morgan spots	Bright red spots Most prominent on the trunk.	Well patient. Do not blanch on pressure, are slightly raised.	Patient does not normally complain, usually an incidental finding associated with aging skin in some populations.

Patients with bleeding history or skin bruising who do not have thrombocytopenia may have an underlying coagulation disorder.

Interpreting Laboratory Tests

Patients with petechiae should have an urgent full blood count and coagulation screen - pro-thrombin time (PT) and activated partial thromboplastin time (APTT) (Table 4).

Table 4. Useful tests in thrombocytopenia

• Blood film • Coagulation screen • Urea and electrolytes • Blood group +/- cross match • B12 and folate • Viral screen • ANF and RhF • Other autoantibodies as clinically indicated
Tests which are commonly requested but not needed in uncomplicated ITP (isolated low platelet count)
• Bone marrow aspiration • Specific platelet auto-antibodies

Table 5. Labspot

– What a blood count can tell you in the emergency situation

Useful blood film features in the emergency situation	Interpretation
Large platelets.	Reactive – consistent with ITP.
Very large platelets (as big as red blood cells).	Indicative of familial thrombocytopathy – e.g Glanzmann's or Bernard Soulier syndromes.
Red cell fragments.	Consider Haemolytic Uraemic syndrome or TTP if clinical situation suggests. Possible DIC if coagulation also abnormal.
Blasts.	Consider leukaemia. Blasts may also be present in leukoerythroblastic blood films.
Hypersegmented neutrophils	B12 deficiency (folate deficiency).
Hypogranular neutrophils	Myelodysplasia

Table 6. Common causes of Thrombocytopenia

With the exception of ITP, the platelet count is usually only mildly decreased.

Common causes of thrombocytopenia	How you might suspect or confirm the cause
Immune thrombocytopenia (ITP)	Platelet count is frequently <$10x10^9$/l. Usually <$20x10^9$/l. Marrow sample is usually not required if blood film normal.
Viraemia	Symptoms or history of viral infection. Serology may be useful. Consider HIV infection if there are risk factors. ITP is rare in men.
Drugs: Illicit drugs Prescription drugs Alternative medicines (e.g Echinacea)	Counts usually mildly low or just outside normal range. Platelet count may have been recorded as normal prior to commencing suspected drug.
Artefactual	The laboratory may notice clumping on the blood film (occurs when platelets stick together). Sending the sample in an alternative anticoagulant (citrate) may allow an accurate count.
Gestational thrombocytopenia	Patient is pregnant. Thrombocytopenia is mild. There is no abnormal bleeding. If the patient has petechiae and a low platelet count, the cause is not gestational thrombocytopenia.

Putting the history, examination and laboratory findings together is essential for making the correct diagnosis in a patient with a thrombocytopenic rash.

Isolated Low Platelet Count-Recommended Investigations

Abrupt onset of petechiae (for example over-night), is typically associated with platelet counts of less than 20 x 10^9/l. Patients with an immune cause for low platelet counts are usually well apart from the petechial rash or mucosal bleeding. The differential diagnosis of a petechial rash includes meningococcal septicaemia, pneumococcal or other septicaemia and Disseminated Intra-Vascular Coagulation (DIC) (Table 7). These patients are usually extremely unwell with disturbance of pulse, BP and temperature, and have coagulation abnormalities consistent with Disseminated Intra-vascular Coagulation.

Patients with a normal platelet count and/or mucosal bleeding may have Von Willebrand's disease, in which endothelial coagulation is disrupted due to the lack or malfunction of Von Willebrand factor. A rare type of Von Willebrand disease (type IIb) has associated thrombocytopenia. The algorithm in figure 5 covers some of the "decision crossroads" commonly encountered when interpreting clinical and laboratory data.

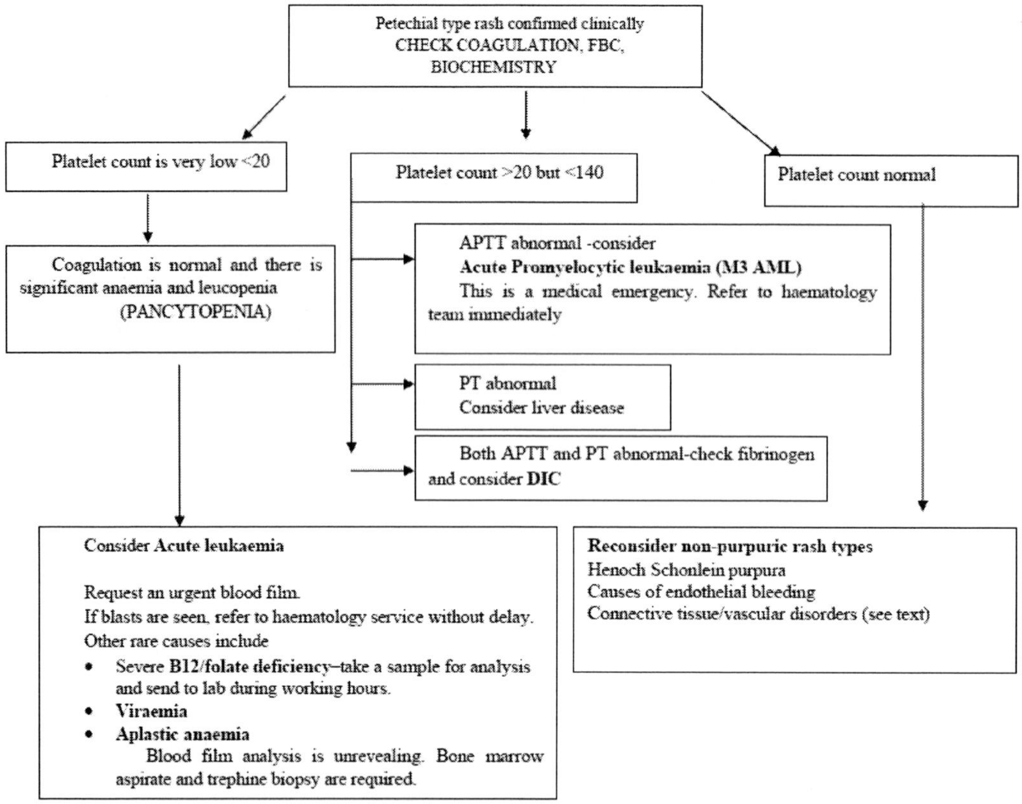

Figure 5. Acute Petechial-type Rash - Decision Tree Analysis.

Table 7. Pearls and Pitfalls -rare but serious causes of thrombocytopenia

Complications may occur if the diagnosis is delayed.

"Worst case" causes of thrombocytopenia	**Clues to these causes**
Meningococcal septicaemia -the most important diagnosis to consider and promptly diagnose	Fever, rapidly changing clinical picture, rash spreading over hours. Rash worse on digits and extremities. Altered level of consciousness, headache, neck stiffness. ANY ONE of these signs should prompt consideration of meningococcal sepsis.
Acute leukaemia (myeloblastic or lymphoblastic)	Usually abnormal haemoglobin and/or white cell count. Sometimes white cell count raised. Usually have blasts in the blood film (although numbers may be low).
Thrombotic thrombocytopenic purpura	Impaired neurological and renal function, fever and microangiopathic haemolytic anaemia.
Haemolytic Uraemic syndrome	History of infection (often gastroenteritis). Bloody diarrhoea. Renal impairment.

"Worst case" causes of thrombocytopenia	**Clues to these causes**
Aplastic anaemia	Anaemia and leucopenia (neutrophils $<1x10^9/l$)
Heparin Induced Thrombocytopenia	Must have had prior heparin exposure – painstaking history-taking is needed to confirm exposure to heparin including heparin flushes. Previous medical records should be requested. Patient may have rapidly developing small vessel thrombosis –most obvious in the extremities.
Disseminated Intravascular Coagulation	Generally occurs in sick hospital inpatients. All aspects of the coagulation screen are abnormal

The recipe for perpetual ignorance is: be satisfied with your opinions and content with your knowledge.

Elbert Hubbard (US Author 1856 – 1915)

In: Learning Clinical Skills
Editors: Bridget Maher and Pat Henn

ISBN: 978-1-62100-409-7

Chapter VII

Meningococcal Septicaemia in Children

Jackelina Pando-Kelly and Deirdre Murray

Clinical Case 1

A seven year old boy is brought to the Emergency Department by his parents. He had been unwell the night before with a raised temperature and painful legs. He had vomited once before bedtime. The following morning at 6a.m. his parents found him pale and mottled with a non-blanching petechial rash on his lower limbs and trunk (Figure 1).

On arrival at the hospital, he was agitated and unwell with cold peripheries. His heart rate was 140 beats per minute, with a capillary refill time of 6 seconds and Oxygen saturations of 92%. His rash progressed rapidly with the development of purpura on both lower limbs. He received 40mls/kg of 0.9% saline and was transferred to the Intensive Care Unit for observation. He was commenced on intravenous Ceftriaxone.

Clinical Case 2

A short while later, the boy's older sister was brought to the Emergency Department by her aunt to be assessed as she was also unwell. On arrival, she was alert, but slightly pale with a capillary refill time of 4 seconds and 3-4 small (1mm) petechiae on her lower limbs. She was commenced on intravenous antibiotics and given a 20ml/kg intravenous bolus of 0.9% saline. Within 30 minutes, she became increasingly agitated and less responsive. Her Glasgow Coma Scale rapidly reduced from 15 to 8 and she required intubation by rapid sequence induction. She was given intravenous mannitol and transferred to the Intensive Care Unit. Her pupillary size returned to normal. CT brain confirmed cerebral oedema. Her fluid intake was restricted and within 48 hours she was extubated and transferred back to the paediatric ward.

With aggressive management, both children began to improve after 24 hours and both made a full recovery after 7 days of intravenous antibiotics.

Diagnosis: Both of these children had invasive meningococcal infection.

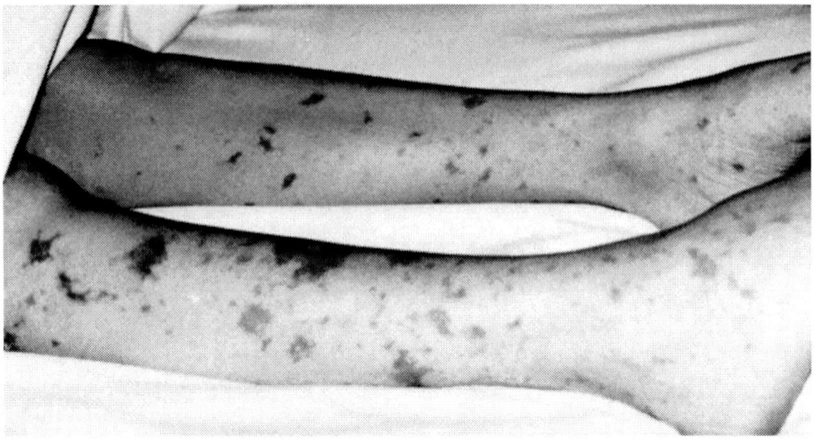

Figure 1. Purpuric rash in Meningococcal Septicaemia.

Discussion

These cases illustrate that meningococcal disease may take the form of meningitis and/or septicaemia. The prognosis is worse with meningococcal septicaemia. Both children were acutely unwell and needed immediately resuscitation. The mortality of meningococcal disease is significant (10% in industrialized countries and higher elsewhere) but with aggressive management, can be decreased significantly.

Meningococcal Disease

Microbiology and Epidemiology

Neisseria meningitides is a common bacterial commensal of the human upper respiratory tract, but it can also become a devastating human pathogen. Meningococci are gram-negative diploccocci and can be encapsulated or unencapsulated. They can cause world wide epidemic meningitis and rapidly progressing fatal shock.

Meningococcal disease can vary in incidence from very rare to over 1000 cases per 100,000 population every year *[1]*. It is more common in children < 5 years of age and in young adults between 15 and 24 years. Meningococcal infection is the most common infectious cause of death in the UK.

Pathophysiology

Acquisition of meningococci through very close contact with respiratory secretions or saliva can be transient, lead to colonisation (carriage), or result in invasive disease.

Absence of protective bactericidal antibodies is the most important single predisposing factor for systemic meningococcal disease. There is an increased risk of recurrent meningococcal infections in individuals with defects in the terminal complement pathway (C5-C9). *[1]*

Endotoxin (lipid A) released from the outer membrane of the bacteria mediates the disease process and is associated with release of several cytokines, chemokines (tumour necrosis factor α, interleukin 1, 6 and 8) and nitric oxide. These lead to diffuse vasculitis, disseminated intravascular coagulation (DIC) and involvement of multiple systems. The level of endotoxin is up to 100 -fold greater in meningococcal septicaemia than in other Gram-negative infections and correlates with mortality.

Table 1. Spectrum of presentation in invasive meningococcal disease

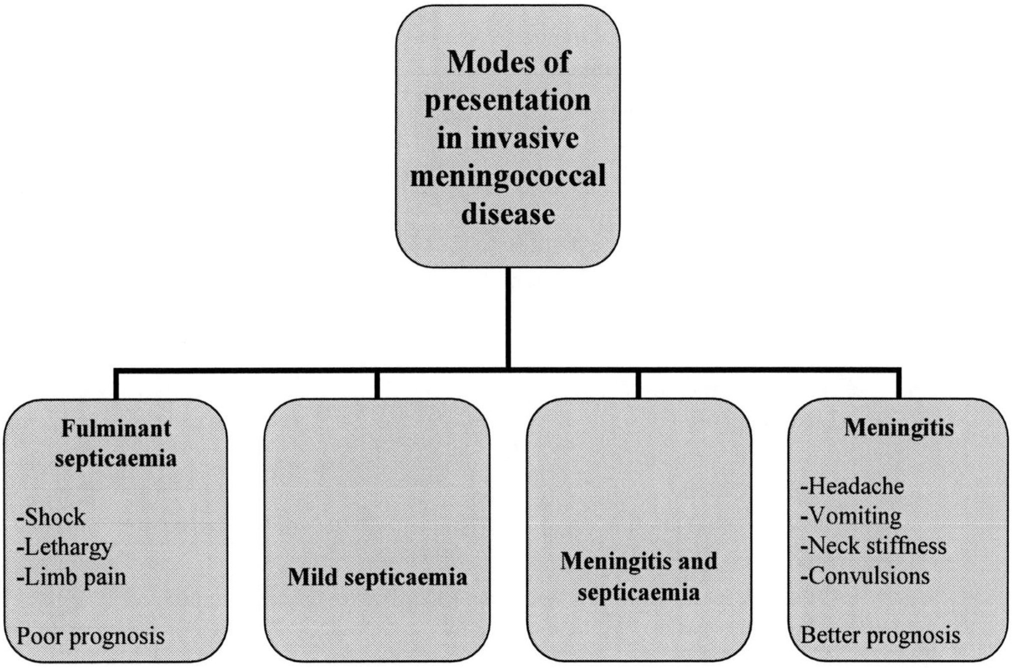

- The mortality rate in septicaemia associated with shock is 20-30%. However, with aggressive management this mortality can be brought down to 2-3%.
- Unlike other causes of bacterial meningitis (i.e. *Streptococcus pneumoniae*), neurological morbidity after meningococcal meningitis is low.
- Early signs may be non-specific: cold extremities, limb pain. These features often precede the appearance of the petechial rash. [3]

Table 2. Causes of Petechial and/or Purpuric rash in children

- **Infection**
  - Neisseria meningitides
  - Group A Streptococcus
  - Streptococcus pneumonia
  - Parvovirus, Adenovirus, Enterovirus
  - Varicella
  - Rickettsia
  - Congenital Infections:TORCH
- **Vasculitis**
  - Henoch-Shönlein Purpura
  - Drug induced
- **Immune**/idiopathic thrombocytopenic purpura
  Hemolytic Uremic Syndrome
- **Disseminated intravascular coagulation**
- **Malignancy**
  - Leukaemia/ lymphoma
- Neonatal alloimmune thrombocytopenia
- **Sequestration / Splenomegaly**
  - Portal Hypertension
  - Storage disease
  - Large hemangiomas(Kasabach Meritt Syndrome)
- **Platelet function abnormalities**
  - Bernard Soulier Syndrome,
  - Medications (aspirin/ibuprofen)
- **Clotting factor disorders**
  - Haemophilia
  - Von Willebrand disease
- Liver disease
- Vitamin K deficiency
- Vitamin C deficiency
  - Neonatal purpura fulminans (congenital Vit C deficiency)
- Ehlers-Danlos Syndrome
- **Other:** forceful vomiting, coughing (distribution usually around face/neck)

Pearls

Remember that in the case of a sick child, you must act immediately, so don't lose time taking a detailed history. You can do this once the child is stable.

Start with:

Physical Examination - Must Check!

You need to identify straight away if the child is seriously ill or not and you will know that by assessing:

- *Level of consciousness.*

  Is the child alert and playful? Or is he lethargic and difficult to arouse? Is he irritable and difficult to console, even by mum? Remember to assess the child's Glasgow meningococcal septicaemia prognostic score (Table 10).
- *Capillary refill time (CRT) and heart rate (HR)*

  In children, CRT and HR are the quickest ways to clinically assess overall perfusion. A prolonged CRT (>2 seconds) and tachycardia are early signs of inadequate cardiac output.

  Hypotension is a very late sign in a child, so do not wait for it. Act to improve circulation if there is tachycardia and prolonged CRT.
- *Distribution* of the rash can be helpful. A small number of petechiae in the distribution of the Superior Vena Cava (upper chest, head and neck) can occur with forceful vomiting or coughing. Think of this especially if the petechiae are only seen around the eyes (periorbital). Diffuse petechiae in a sick child makes the diagnosis of meningococcal disease more likely.
- The *size* of the petechiae is also helpful. If greater than 1-2 mm diameter they are described as purpura and more likely to be due to meningococcal disease in a sick child.

History– Must Ask!

- Early symptoms and signs: fever, generally unwell, muscle ache/joint pain, especially of lower limbs.
- Ask about sick contacts.

Lab Spot

Recommended investigations in an unwell child with decreased level of consciousness (LOC) and petechial/purpuric rash (Table 4).

Management of Meningococcal Septicaemia

Management of acute septic shock in children is different from that of adults. Children require greater amounts of fluid resuscitation and are more likely to require inotropic support.

Principles of Management of Meningococcal Septicaemia/Septic Shock

1. ABC

   A: Airway: Make sure that the child's airway is patent.
   You may need to use an oral or nasopharyngeal airway, or perform an airway opening manoeuvre in an unconscious child.

   B: Breathing: If child is not breathing spontaneously, bag–mask ventilation should be started until endotracheal intubation and mechanical ventilation is provided.

   C: Circulation: If peripheral pulses are not palpable and/or the capillary refill time is prolonged, aggressive fluid replacement to maintain perfusion to vital organs is needed.

If there is persistent evidence of poor perfusion in spite of fluid replacement (60mls/kg), then inotropes should be commenced, and the child should be transferred to the Intensive Care Unit.

2. *Antibiotics* should be given as soon as possible. In a primary care setting, this should take the form of intramuscular Benzylpenicillin. In the hospital setting, your choice should be 3rd generation cephalosporin.
3. Continuous *assessment* with Glasgow Meningococcal Septicaemia Prognostic Score and *monitoring* of vital signs. Transfer to ICU if needed.
4. *Treatment of coagulopathy* to reduce complications of liver and kidney failure, life-threatening haemorrhage and peripheral limb loss. You may need to give transfusions of packed red blood cells, fresh frozen plasma and/or cryoprecipitate.
5. Reduce *skin, soft tissue and skeletal complications* such as significant necrosis and bone ischemia. May need fasciotomies, grafting, and/or amputation.

Remember to look for and treat:

- Acidosis
- Anaemia
- Hypoglycaemia
- Hypokalemia
- Hypocalcemia
- Hypomagnesaemia

Prophylaxis

Neisseria meningitides tends to colonize the nasopharynx, so an asymptomatic carrier state is common. All household members and close contacts should receive chemoprophylaxis to prevent secondary cases. The antibiotic of choice is oral rifampicin

Table 3. Causes of decreased level of consciousness in children

• *Infections* - Septic shock - Bacterial meningitis - Viral encephalitis - Post infectious encephalomyelitis • *Dehydration/Hypotension* • *Metabolic disturbances* - Hypoglycemia - Diabetic ketoacidosis -I nborn errors of metabolism - Electrolyte imbalance - Addisonian crisis • *Neurological disorders* - Seizures - Raised intracranial pressure:Hydrocephalus, brain tumour - Cerebrovascular accident - Hypertensive encephalopathy • *Respiratory failure* • *Cardiac* - Heart failure - Arrhythmia - Myocardial infarction • *Trauma* • *Medications* • *Overdose/ Poisoning* • *Toxic:* alcohol ingestion, drugs • *Post chemotherapy* • *Psychiatric:* catatonia

Table 4. Unwell child with decreased LOC and petechial/purpuric rash -Investigations

• Full blood count and differential • Blood glucose • Urea and electrolytes • Coagulation screen • Liver function tests • C-reactive protein • Blood cultures • Arterial or venous blood gases • Serum meningococcal and pneumococcal PCR • Urine microscopy and culture • Throat swab • Lumbar puncture (LP)[*] • CT/MRI [2]

Table 4. (Continued)

* A lumbar puncture should be deferred in the presence of:

1. Shock.
2. Coagulopathy.
3. Raised intracranial pressure.

A child with meningococcal disease may have all three, and so empirical antibiotic therapy is appropriate, with the LP deferred until the child is clinically stable (Table 5).

[2] If persistent decrease in LOC, seizures, suspicion of increased intracranial pressure (ICP) or focal neurological signs. Imaging may be indicated if the child continues to have persistent fever following several days of antibiotics, as the formation of a subdural abscess is a possibility.

Table 5. Contraindications to performing a lumbar puncture in children with suspected meningitis

- Signs suggesting raised ICP:
  - ↓ or fluctuating LOC
  - bradycardia and hypertension
  - focal neurological signs
  - abnormal posture or posturing
  - unequal, dilated or poorly responsive pupils
  - papilloedema
- Shock
- Extensive or spreading purpura
- After seizures (until stabilized)
- Coagulation abnormalities
- Local superficial infection at the LP site
- Respiratory insufficiency

Table 6. Fluid Management in Septic Shock in Children

- Bolus of Sodium Chloride (0.9%)
  20ml/kg over 5-10 minutes -can repeat up to 3 times.
- If no improvement in perfusion after 60mls/kg- consider inotropes.

Table 7. Antibiotics in Suspected Meningococcal Septicaemia

- 3rd generation cephalosporin. Ceftriaxone or Cefotaxime IV.
- If no IV access: Benzylpenicillin IM
  - 1-9 years: 600mg
  - >9 years and adults: 1.2g
- Antibiotics should be continued for at least 7 days.

Table 8. Treatment of Coagulopathy

- Fresh frozen plasma, platelets, cryoprecipitate
- Vitamin K
- Avoid intramuscular injections

Table 9. Co-existent meningitis –Pearls

Watch for signs of raised intracranial pressure: decreasing level of consciousness, abnormal posturing, unequal pupillary signs.

- Avoid fluid overload.
- Intravenous mannitol.
- Head of bed elevated to 30°.

Table 10. Glasgow Meningococcal Septicaemia Prognostic Score

D. GLASGOW MENINGOCOCCAL SEPTICAEMIA PROGNOSTIC SCORE

The Glasgow Meningococcal Septicaemia Prognostic Score (GMSPS) is composed of 7 parts, 6 clinical and 1 laboratory value. It is described below.

Observation	Score
BP <75 mmHg age <4 <85 mmHg age ≥4	3
Skin / rectal temp difference >3	3
Modified coma score <8 or deterioration of 3 points or more in 1hr	3
Deterioration in 1 hour before scoring	2
Absence of meningism	2
Extending purpuric rash or widespread purpura	1
Base deficit > 8	1
Maximum total score	15

A score > 8 indicates a poor outcome.
Reproduced by kind permission of the Meningitis Research Foundation. www.meningitisUK.org.

Pitfalls

- Some children with meningococcal infection will present primarily with non-specific symptoms or signs and may be difficult to distinguish from other less important (viral) infections with a similar presentation.*[2]*
- Classical signs of meningitis (neck stiffness, photophobia, high-pitched cry) are often absent in infants with bacterial meningitis.*[2]* A bulging fontanelle is a late sign.
- A rash may be less visible in darker skin tone children, so remember to check soles, palms and conjunctivae.
- A small number of petechiae in an unwell child does not rule out meningococcal disease (see note on distribution).
- Do not wait too long between fluid boluses to assess response. Once the bolus has been given, perfusion should improve. If no improvement occurs, move quickly to next bolus and/or inotropes.
- Defer doing an LP in a very sick child until the child is stable.
- Early treatment of coagulation abnormalities in meningococcal disease is important in order to prevent complications.

Tips for the OSCE

- Even in an emergency, and when dealing with a sick child, you should always be courteous and polite to mum and gentle with the child.
- You must always check the peripheral pulses in a sick child. If they are weak and/or difficult to palpate, and accompanied by tachycardia and prolonged CRT, the child may be in shock.
- Always seek senior advice when dealing with a sick child.
- Remember -Teamwork!
- The initial management in a sick child, regardless of the cause, is always the same: *ABC* and *D*on't Ever *F*orget the *G*lucose.
- When suspecting meningococcal disease, consider other non-specific features of the child's presentation, such as:
  - Level of parental concern (particularly compared with previous illness).
  - How quickly the illness is progressing, *and*
  - Clinical judgement of the overall severity of the illness.

Student Check List

- How do you assess perfusion in a child?
- What is the difference between petechiae and purpura?
- What is Cushing's triad?
- What are the meningococcal serotypes that cause invasive disease?
- Which are the features in meningococcal disease associated with a poor prognosis?
- What is Waterhouse-Friederichsen syndrome?

It Happened to me

In my first registrar post, I was called to a two year boy with a rapidly progressing purpuric rash. He was mottled with a CRT of 6-8 seconds and was agitated. He received a fluid bolus and intravenous antibiotics. The anaesthetic team was called.

As he was not hypotensive, the decision was made to give a further fluid bolus and observe. He soon became less responsive and we rapidly proceeded to intubation. During intubation he became bradycardic and required cardio-pulmonary massage. In retrospect, this boy needed more aggressive fluid resuscitation. The anaesthetic given for intubation caused vasodilation and reduced his venous return and preload, dropping his cardiac output and leading to bradycardia.

Table 11. Age-specific frequency of clinical features of meningococcal disease prior to hospital admission

	<1 year %	1 to 4 years %	5 to 14 years %	15 to 16 years %
Early features				
Leg pain	5.1	30.6	62.4	53.3
Thirst	3.4	6.4	11.4	12.6
Diarrhoea	9.9	7.8	3.1	5.5
Abnormal colour	20.6	16.8	18.5	19.0
Breathing difficulty	16.2	9.7	7.1	12.1
Cold extremities	44.0	46.7	34.9	44.4
'Classic' features				
Haemorrhagic rash	42.3	64.2	69.8	65.9
Neck pain or stiffness	15.5	28.1	45.9	52.9
Photophobia	24.5	24.1	26.4	35.5
Bulging fontanelle	11.5	n/a	n/a	n/a
Late features				
Confusion or delirium	n/a	42.8	49.4	47.6
Seizure	8.9	12.8	7.8	7.3
Unconscious	7.0	9.1	5.9	15.1

Table reproduced with permission from the Lancet (Thompson et al 2006 [3]).

Remember:

- A child can be in shock, even with a normal blood pressure.
- Quick and aggressive management of shock in meningococcal disease is a life saving measure.

Observe, record, tabulate, communicate. Use your five senses. ... Learn to see, learn to hear, learn to feel, learn to smell, and know that by practice alone you can become expert.

Sir William Osler

References

[1] Stephens DS, Greenwood B, Brandtzaeg P. Epidemic meningitis, meningococcaemia, and *Neisseria meningitides. Lancet* 2007; 369:2196-210

[2] National Institute for Health and Clinical Excellence (NICE) clinical guideline 102 Developed by the National Collaborating Centre for Women's and Children's Health. Bacterial meningitis and meningococcal septicaemia Management of bacterial meningitis and meningococcal septicaemia in children and young people younger than 16 years in primary and secondary care. Issue date: June 2010, revised September 2010.

[3] Thompson MJ, Ninis N, Perera R, Levin M. Clinical recognition of meningococcal disease in children and adolescents. *Lancet.* Feb 2006;367(9508):397-403.

Recommended Reading

Bilukha O.O, Rosenstein N. Prevention and control of meningococcal disease: recommendations of the Advisory Committee on Immunization Practices (ACIP). *MMWR Morb Mortal Wkly Rep* 2005; 54(RR-7):1.

In: Learning Clinical Skills
Editors: Bridget Maher and Pat Henn
ISBN: 978-1-62100-409-7

Chapter VIII

Neonatal Jaundice and the Newborn Screening Examination

Tony Ryan

Clinical Case

A midwife on the postnatal ward contacts you expressing concern about a newborn male infant in her care. Having identified herself, she gives you an SBAR (Situation, Background, Assessment, Recommendation) handover account. The *situation* is that she measured a transcutaneous bilirubin (TcBili) on the 36-hour baby who appeared clinically jaundiced and found it to read 270mmol/L. The *background* was that the baby was born normally, at term, to healthy parents, with a birth weight of 3.6 kg and a current weight of 3.4 kg. There was no prolonged rupture of the membranes. Mum is breastfeeding and while her milk supply is not yet flourishing, it is progressing well. The baby is having transitional stools, and is latching on and sucking well. The baby appears contented and is not listless. The mother's blood group is O positive. The midwife's *assessment* is that this most likely represents physiological jaundice. Her *recommendation* is that a serum bilirubin is warranted, since the TcBilirubin is just a screening tool and, in general, tends to underestimate the actual serum bilirubin. She also notes that the baby has not had a newborn screening examination (NSE).

Discussion

Reflection before Action: Experts think by intuition (pattern recognition) along with metacognition (a combination of emotional intelligence, analytical thinking, clinical reasoning, strategic planning and motivation to learn). As a novice doctor, with limited practical experience, your pattern recognition skills in neonatology are still limited. Unlike the expert who is on autopilot as he makes his way to see baby, you feel nervous and uncertain. Therefore you need to start regulating your emotions (you take a deep breath) and start concentrating on your thinking (metacognition) - what do you expect to hear, see and discover upon arrival? If you can work out the main 3-5 possible diagnoses of neonatal jaundice, you can prepare a line of questioning within a definite line of reasoning and perform a more focused and purposeful examination of the baby. This approach (hypothesis-led clinical examination) has been shown to increase diagnostic ability among student doctors. In contrast, interviewing behaviors characteristic of poorly rated diagnosticians included repeating questions unnecessarily, changing the topic before completing a line of inquiry and inquiring about past history during the first three minutes of the consultation. [1]

Neonatal jaundice is extremely common - 50-60% of newborn infants become jaundiced during the first week of life. You consider the causes of jaundice in the newborn (Table 1) along with the information provided by the midwife. From her assessment, this baby is not likely to be sick and there are no risk factors for infection, probably excluding sepsis as the cause of this baby's jaundice.

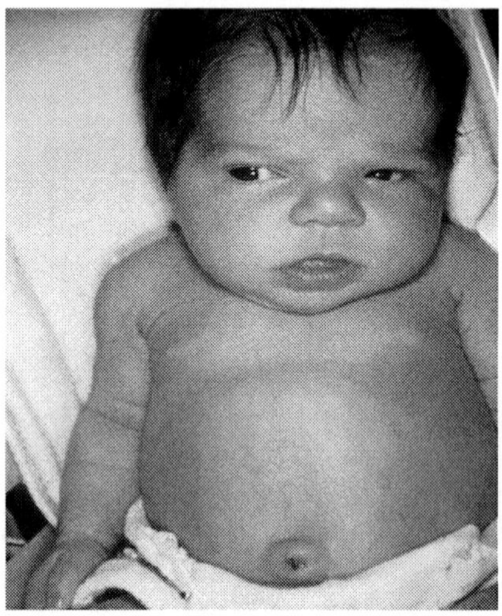

Figure 1. A jaundiced baby. (Incidentally, the coarse facies, protruding tongue, distended abdomen and umbilical hernia in this particular baby suggest a diagnosis of congenital hypothyroidism).

Table 1. Causes of Jaundice in the early neonatal period

- Physiological
- Breast feeding (hypernatraemic dehydration)
- Maternal-foetal blood group incompatibility
- Sepsis
- Polycythaemia
- Cephalohematoma
- Galactosaemia (rare)*
- Congenital Spherocytosis*
- G6PD deficiency*

* Rare causes.

- Healthy newborns commonly become jaundiced because their immature livers are slow to process bilirubin (*physiologic* jaundice).
- Jaundice is also fairly common among *breastfeeding* babies who aren't getting enough milk. Such infants may have excessive weight loss (>10% of birth weight) and elevated serum Na^{+}(>150mmol/l - *hypernatremic dehydration*). However, this diagnosis is unlikely since the baby has lost only 5% of birth weight.
- Neonatal jaundice is also seen in cases of *maternal-fetal blood type incompatibility* where the mother's body produces antibodies that attack the fetus's blood cells. Since the mother's blood group is O positive, Rhesus disease does not apply. However, an ABO incompatibility is possible if the baby has A, B or AB blood type. The baby's blood group and Coombs' test will be useful investigations.
- Another cause of neonatal jaundice is *polycythaemia*, a condition in which a child is born with an excess of red blood cells. It can be diagnosed by clinical examination and confirmed by a full blood count.
- A large scalp *cephalohematoma* can cause jaundice - as the body naturally breaks down this clotted blood, the baby's liver is unable to handle the excess bilirubin released.
- Rarer causes of jaundice include *congenital spherocytosis*: there may be a family history, although some cases occur *de novo*. A blood film can help exclude this condition.
- If the parents are of Asian origin, deficiency of the red cell enzyme, *G6PD*, must also be considered.
- Galactosaemia is an uncommon autosomal recessive condition that is potentially lethal if not diagnosed early. It has an incidence of 1/400 births among the Irish travelling community. A Beutler test for galactosaemia is done on day one of life in these babies.

With the above considerations in mind, examination of the baby will focus on the baby's general condition (exclude sepsis), size (small for dates: congenital infection), skin (petechiae, ecchymoses: the so-called Blueberry Muffin baby with a congenital infection), liver/spleen enlargement (infection or haemolysis with extra-medullary haematopoeisis), eyes (cataracts; congenital infection and galactosaemia). Most mild cases of jaundice resolve spontaneously in a week or so. However, high bilirubin levels can cause hearing loss and brain damage in babies *(kernicterus)*. Because of the decline in Rhesus disease, the current groups at risk for kernicterus in developed countries are breastfeeding, early discharge from hospital and babies with dark skin. Babies with high bilirubin levels may need *phototherapy*, or in rare cases, an *exchange transfusion* (figure 2). Phototherapy causes photodegradation of bilirubin in the infant's skin.

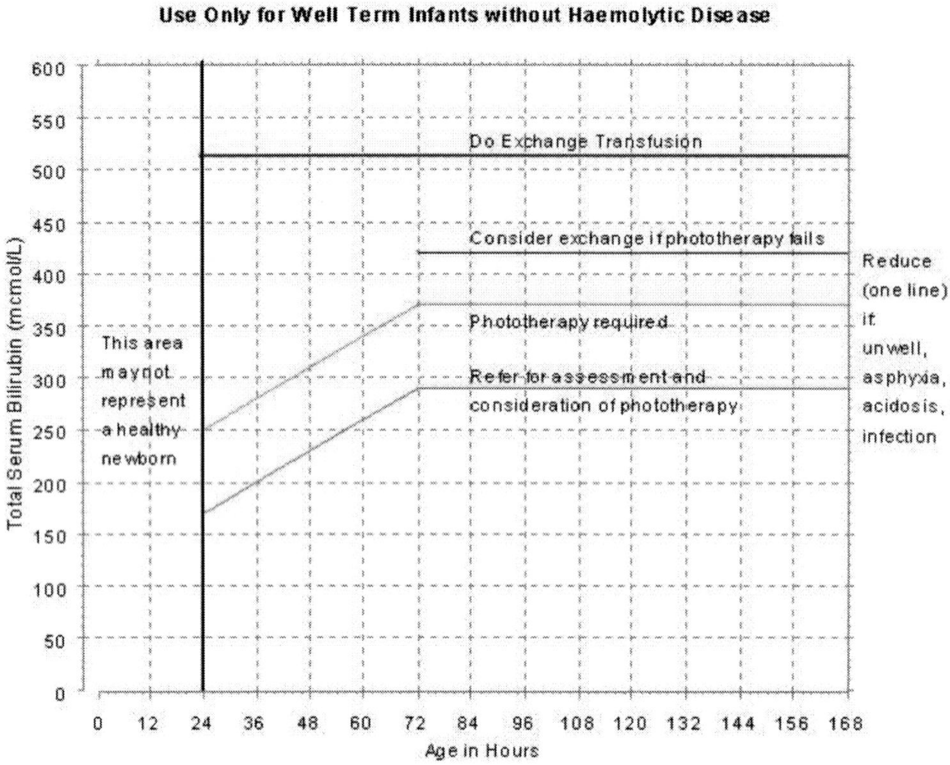

Figure 2. Jaundice Treatment Guidelines for term babies without haemolysis.
Reproduced with kind permission Newborn Services Clinical Guideline, Auckland City Hospital, New Zealand. http://www.adhb.govt.nz/newborn/guidelines/GI/Jaundice.htm.

Table 2. Equipment for the Newborn Screening Examination

- Stethoscope: appropriate size, clean and warm
- Disposable paper measuring tape
- Ophthalmoscope to check the red light reflex
- Torch and tongue depressor for examining the palate
- Patella hammer
- Pulse oximeter to measure lower limb O_2 saturations
- Calibrated Transcutaneous Bilirubinometer
- 25% oral sucrose solution for analgesia during blood sampling
- Capillary blood sampling equipment and gloves
- Consent form to permit baby to be screened for sensori-neural hearing loss; incidence 1-2 per 1000 births
- Warm hands

Here is a possible checklist for your meeting with the parents (Table 3).

Table 3. General Approach

- Ask permission to enter the room; wait for an answer.
- Introduce yourself, showing ID badge.
- Wash your hands.
- Sit down. Smile if appropriate.
- Ask for the baby's name and gender.
- Review the antenatal history, antenatal screening, family history, pregnancy and labor and address any relevant issues with parents.
- Follow a logical line of inquiry in relationship to the baby's jaundice.
- Do a review of the parent's perspective (RPP).
- Encourage maternal support of baby during the examination (Figure 3).
- *A review of parent perspectives (RPP):* You are thinking about the parents. This is their first baby and naturally enough they will be concerned and anxious. You want to show them that you value their insights and contribution by sitting down and giving them time to openly express their concerns by asking them: 'What are your biggest worries about your baby?' You also assess their *prior knowledge* and *understanding* of neonatal jaundice: 'What have you been told about your baby's condition?' and 'what do you understand about your baby's condition?
- *Hand-swaddling the baby:* You show the mother how she can help during the physical examination (figure 3) by containing and comforting her baby, supportive techniques that have recently been shown to reduce crying in infants undergoing NSE [2].

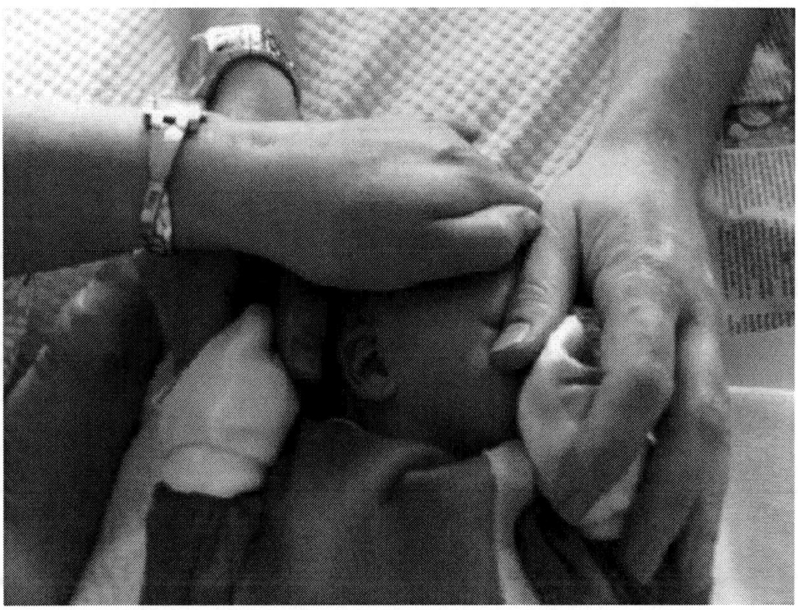

Figure 3. A mother supporting and containing her baby by hand-swaddling.

The Newborn Screening Examination

- The NSE [3,4] is a standardized examination performed on every newborn infant. It aims to identify potentially correctable defects that may interfere with normal development. The NSE includes an examination for size, macrocephaly or microcephaly, changes in skin color, signs of birth trauma, malformations, evidence of respiratory distress, level of arousal, posture, tone, presence of spontaneous movements, and symmetry of movement. A careful examination helps the physician to detect anomalies, birth injuries, and cardiorespiratory disorders that may compromise a newborn's successful adaptation to extrauterine life.
- The approach and order to the NSE varies among individual doctors. Most of the NSE is by observation of baby's features, activity, color and by counting the infant's respiratory rate.
- A head to toe scanning for congenital anomalies, including auscultation of the heart to exclude murmurs, then follows.
- Having a standard systematic approach to the examination of the infant makes it less likely that any essential part of the examination is omitted. However, your routine should be flexible and opportunistic. If the infant is quiet and relaxed when first approached, auscultation of the heart and palpation of the abdomen should precede more disturbing examinations such as examination of the mouth and hips.
- Practice "thinking out-loud" as you perform the NSE. You will find that babies are soothed and parents are reassured by a continuous low tone commentary ("nice heart... nice tummy...beautiful baby..."). If you note a clinical problem, it's best to acknowledge it to the parents: "I am not completely happy with the baby's left hip, but I will talk to you about it when the examination is complete".

Approaching the Examination – Check-List

Be familiar with the normal range of neonatal parameters (Table 4). The baby's *weight*, crown-heel *length*, and *head circumference* should be plotted on the appropriate centile chart, as all parameters of growth need to be related to gestational age and gender for interpretation.

Table 4. Normal Neonatal values

- Respiratory rate: 40-60/min
- Heart rate :120-160/min
- Head circumference at term (33-38 cm)
- Low birth weight = < 2500 gm

Cover, Color, Count

Cover: Observe the baby's features looking for any obvious malformations or dysmorphism, position, activity, nutritional status, birthmarks, body proportions, fingers and toes. Are there any obvious malformations? In particular, is the baby unusual-looking, e.g. Down syndrome? If the infant is small for dates or unusually thin, look for signs of fetal malnutrition, such as dry scaly skin on the abdomen and extremities and/or abdominal skin creases and lack of normal subcutaneous fat. These babies need to be watched for hypoglycaemia and fed early. Large for date's babies may follow maternal gestational diabetes and also require close glucose monitoring. Erythematic toxic neonatorum (figure 4, below), transient neonatal pustular melanosis, sucking blister, miliaria, neonatal acne and Mongolian spots are among the many benign skin conditions that can occur in newborns.

Color: Note whether the baby is generally plethoric or pale, pink or blue in the mouth and lips, or if the baby is jaundiced. Blue hands and feet are normal features in an otherwise well baby.

Count: Count the respiratory rate noting that an irregular breathing pattern is normal. You are not likely to find a respiratory diagnosis if the respiratory rate is normal. Listen for a grunt (on expiration) or a stridor (on inspiration).

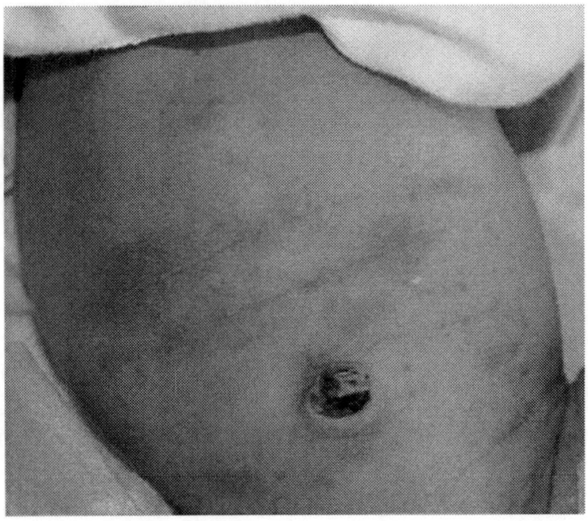

Figure 4. Erythema toxicum.
Erythema toxicum is a common and completely benign condition seen in about half of healthy infants in the first 2 days of life.

Head and Neck Examination

- Note the size, shape and lie of the baby's head.
- Measure the maximum head circumference to diagnose macrocephaly or microcephaly.
- Feel the anterior fontanelle for signs of tension and/or separation of the suture lines.

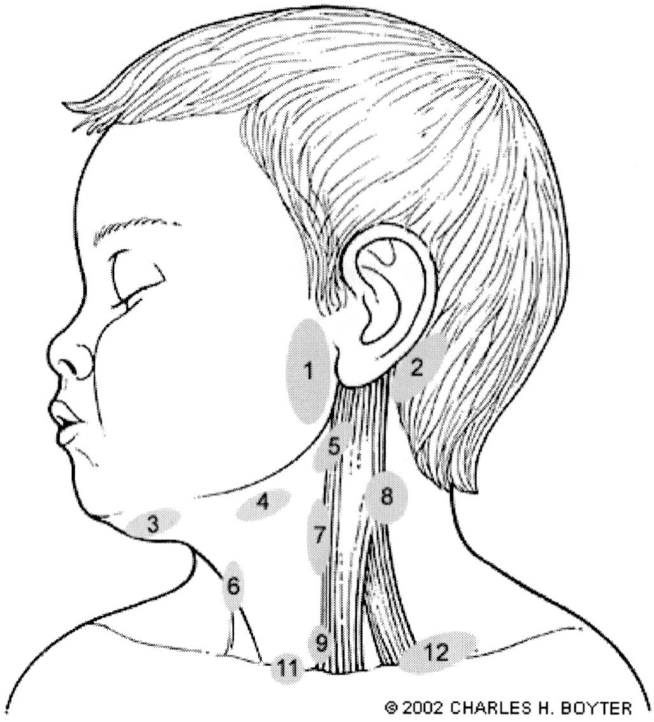

Figure 5. Congenital neck masses by location [3, 5]. Reproduced by kind permission of the American Academy of Family Physicians. Fuloria M, Kreiter S. The Newborn Examination: Part I. American Family Physician. 2002. Jan 1;65(1):61-69.

1 = Preauricular area (parotid gland): congenital lesions-cystic hygroma, hemangioma, venous malformation; inflammatory condition-lymphadenitis secondary to infection in upper face and/or anterior scalp.

2 = Postauricular area: congenital lesions-branchial cleft I (cystic, inflamed, or both); inflammatory condition-lymphadenitis secondary to inflammation of posterior scalp.

3 = Submental area: congenital lesions-thyroglossal duct cyst, cystic hygroma, dermoid cyst, venous malformation; inflammatory condition-lymphadenitis secondary to inflammation in perioral area, anterior oral area, or nasal cavity.

4 =Submandibular area: congenital lesions-cystic hygroma, hemangioma, ranula; inflammatory condition-lymphadenitis of submandibular gland secondary to inflammation in cheek and/or mid-oral cavity; in cystic fibrosis, enlargement of submandibular gland without inflammation.

5 = Jugulodiagastric area (tonsil node; normal structures include transverse process of C2 and styloid process): congenital lesions-branchial cleft I or II, hemangioma, cystic hygroma; inflammatory condition-lymphadenitis secondary to oropharyngeal inflammation.

6 = Area of neck midline (normal structures include hyoid, thyroid isthmus, and thyroid cartilage): congenital lesions-thyroglossal duct cyst, dermoid cyst; inflammatory condition-lymphadenitis.

7 = Area at anterior border of sternocleidomastoid muscle (normal structures include hyoid, thyroid cartilage, and carotid bulb): congenital lesions-branchial cleft I, II, or III (IV is rare), laryngocele, hemangioma, lymphangioma, hematoma (fibroma of sternocleidomastoid muscle).

8 = Spinal accessory: inflammatory condition-lymphadenitis secondary to nasopharyngeal inflammation. 9. Paratracheal area: thyroid mass, parathyroid mass, esophageal diverticulum, metastatic lesion. 10=Supraclavicular area (normal structures include fat pad, pneumatocele from apical lobe related to defect in Gibson fascia [prominent mass with Valsalva's maneuver]): congenital lesion-cystic hygroma; neoplastic lesion-lipoma. 11= Suprasternal area: thyroid mass, lipoma, dermoid cyst, thymus mass, mediastinal mass.

- Look for caput succedaneum, cephalohematoma (usually benign and does not cross the midline) or subgaleal hemorrhage (a boggy swelling crossing the midline posteriorly). This can be a lethal hemorrhage as the subgaleal space can accommodate the baby's total blood volume (80 ml/kg).
- Feel the bridge of the nose for septal deviation.
- Note that the eyes and ears are normally shaped and placed.
- Use an ophthalmoscope to see that the red reflex shows no central black spots (cataracts), dullness or irregularities (glaucoma), or white reflex (retinoblastoma).
- Subconjunctival hemorrhages are common after vaginal delivery and usually do not represent ocular trauma.
- Conjunctivitis is relatively common in newborns. Think of possible STI causes such as gonorrhea or chlamydia, although these are rare.
- Be aware that most facial nerve palsies (usually associated with a forceps delivery) resolve spontaneously.
- Palpate the sternomastoid muscles and the range of rotation of the head to exclude a congenital torticollis.
- Look and feel for a cleft palate, especially if micrognathia present (Pierre Robin sequence).
- Palpate for clavicular fractures, especially in larger neonates.
- Neck masses are rare but can be identified by their location, and include vascular malformations, abnormal lymphatic tissue, teratomas, and dermoid cysts (Figure 5).

Cardio-Respiratory Examination

- You have already counted the baby's respiratory rate.
- Is the baby struggling to breathe? Are there any other signs of respiratory distress (subcostal or intercostal indrawing, nasal flaring or head bobbing)?
- Breathing with the belly (diaphragmatic breathing) and periodic breathing (slow deep breaths followed by rapid shallow periods) are normal in babies.
- Look at and feel the apex to determine if the heart is dynamic or quiet, and confirm that the heart is in the normal position (exclude dextrocardia).
- Listen for murmurs.
- Feel for the peripheral pulses. Diminished pulses in all extremities indicate poor cardiac output or peripheral vasoconstriction. Absent or diminished femoral pulses suggest the presence of ductal-dependent cardiac lesions (e.g. coarctation of the aorta).
- Measure lower limb oxygen saturations. If below 95%, organize a CXR, EKG and an echocardiogram to exclude a respiratory cause or a congenital heart defect.
- Blood pressure is measured in all babies admitted to the Neonatal Unit, but is not usually a routine part of the postnatal NSE.

Examining the Abdomen, Hips, Groin, Perineum, Feet, Spine

- Observe the umbilicus for signs of herniation, inflammation or bleeding.
- Feel the abdomen for abdominal masses (rare) and for kidney, liver or spleen enlargement. A liver edge of 1-2 cm can normally be palpated.
- In boys, confirm that both testes are in the scrotum. Testicular hydrocoeles are common and usually resolve spontaneously.
- Reassure the parents that the foreskin is not normally retractile at birth. If the foreskin is hooded (incomplete), look for signs of hypospadias.
- Perform the Barlow and Ortorlani examinations of the hips to detect instability.
- Note the injection site on the thigh where intramuscular Vitamin K was administered to prevent hemorrhagic disease of the newborn. Oral vitamin K may have alternatively been used.
- Ask whether the baby has passed meconium and note that the anus is patent.
- Examine the position and range of motion of the feet. Where club feet (fixed equino or talipes varus or calcaneo valgus deformities) are present, refer to an orthopaedic surgeon. Positional talipes usually responds to passive movement exercises.
- Look for signs of spinal dysraphism. Blind-ended coccxygeal dimples are common and do not usually require further investigations.

Neurological Examination

- Note whether the baby is asleep, awake, arousable or listless.
- Look at the baby's posture for signs of good muscular tone (flexion of limbs) and symmetry.
- Describe any spontaneous movement of the limbs: if one arm is not moving, consider Erb's palsy or a fracture. This diagnosis is reinforced by an asymmetrical Moro reflex.
- Look for the degree of head lag by carefully bringing the baby up by the hands (traction reflex), while also feeling the strength of the grasp reflex.
- In vertical suspension, the baby should not slip through your hands if tone is normal.
- In ventral suspension, the newborn baby lies in an inverted "U" position.
- Check the tone of the limbs and that the tendon reflexes (patellar are the easiest) are present and symmetrical.
- Measure and chart the head circumference according to gender and gestation.

Conclusion

Physical examination of the baby was normal apart from jaundice. The baby was active and vigorous and did not appear dehydrated or sick. There was no hepato-splenomegaly or signs of a congenital infection (TORCHS: Toxoplasma, Rubella, Cytomegalovirus, Herpes, Syphilis). Since the mother is O positive, you suspect hemolysis due to an ABO incompatibility as the cause of the jaundice.

Table 5. Lab-Spot: Focus on Neonatal Jaundice

- Request infant's blood group and Coombs' test if mother's blood group is O (maternal blood group, Rhesus status and screening for hemolytic antibodies are usually done antenatally).
- Hemoglobin, WBC and differential, and reticulocytes if suspicion or evidence of hemolysis or anemia.
- Blood culture and urine for microscopy and culture if clinical suspicion of infection.
- Check the serum bilirubin (SBR). The significance of the SBR estimation depends upon the maturity and postnatal age of the infant, the clinical status of the infant (hypoxemia, acidemia, hypoalbuminemia, and/or hypothermia) and the etiology of the jaundice (Rhesus incompatibility is usually more aggressive than an ABO incompatibility).
- Serial SBR estimations are an essential component of the continuing assessment and management of the jaundiced newborn infant. Graphs (Figure 2) aid in the interpretation of SBR.

Pitfalls

- Atypical presentation of jaundice (early onset, rapid rise in SBR, prolonged jaundice, and/or late onset jaundice) is likely to reflect pathology.
- Transcutaneous bilirubin should not be used in the first 24 hours of life (since early jaundice is usually pathological and serum bilirubin and other investigations are warranted). It is also not reliable during phototherapy.

Pearls

- Newborn screening examination requires knowledge of the usual and the normal.
- Earliest possible detection of abnormalities is important especially where early diagnosis can be life-saving (e.g. esophageal atresia, imperforate anus, and diaphragmatic hernia) or associated with a better functional outcome (e.g. congenital dislocation of the hips, club feet and cataracts).

- A newborn baby with one anatomic malformation should be evaluated for associated anomalies.
- Newborns with cyanosis should be evaluated expeditiously. Respiratory disease is more likely in newborns who are tachypneic and using accessory muscles of respiration.
- Newborns with heart disease generally breathe normally, except for mild tachypnea.
- Causes of cyanosis in infants include airway disorders (choanal atresia), pulmonary causes (respiratory distress syndrome, pneumonia), cardiac disorders (transposition of the great vessels), abdominal distension (bowel obstruction), central nervous system (e.g. asphyxia), metabolic causes (hypoglycemia), polycythemia and hypothermia.
- In newborns, a murmur does not always signify the presence of heart disease, nor does the absence of a murmur provide reassurance of normality. Newborns with relatively benign lesions, such as small ventricular septal defects, often have the loudest murmurs, whereas newborns with severe heart disease may have no murmurs.
- Soft localized murmurs in the immediate newborn period are usually innocent and represent a transition from fetal to neonatal circulation (ductus arteriosus not fully closed).
- Diminished pulses in all extremities indicate poor cardiac output or peripheral vasoconstriction. Absent or diminished femoral pulses suggest the presence of ductal dependent cardiac lesions (e.g., coarctation of the aorta).
- Bile-stained vomiting in a newborn is an emergency and indicates bowel obstruction until proven otherwise.
- Neonatal blood screening for rare treatable conditions is usually done at 48-72 hours of age to avoid the natural surge in thyroxin at birth (leading to false negatives), and to ensure sufficient protein intake for amino-acid disorders of metabolism (PKU, MSUD and tyrosinemia) to present. However, if galactosemia is suspected, send an immediate blood sample to the regional Newborn Screening Testing Laboratory. The baby should remain on a lactose-free formula until galactosemia is excluded.

Tips for the OSCE

- Diagnostic accuracy is maximized by preparing a rational line of questioning, and linking to potential clinical signs and diagnostic possibilities in advance of the physical examination. Think from the start!
- Be precise, concise and pertinent (relevant).
- Don't assume anything. Test your assumptions by asking the appropriate relevant questions.
- Cover, Color, Count. Be honest and observant. Say what you see, not what you think you see or what you would like to see. *(Sherlock Holmes to a disheartened Dr Watson: The trouble, dear Watson, is that you see, but you do not observe. The distinction is clear).*

- Think out-loud, pointing out the normal and healthy features to the parents (and the examiner).
- Don't jump to conclusions.
- Be prepared to change your mind if new evidence is uncovered.
- Avoid clichés: e.g. "She is moving all four limbs" (when it's obvious she is not). "He is not in any obvious distress". Are you sure? Do you mean respiratory distress or psychological distress?
- Remember RPP: Review of parent perspective (page 5).
- It's best to check the following when the baby is quiet: auscultation of the heart, visualizing the red light reflex, the hip examination, and detection of the femoral pulses.
- Rapid undressing may cause baby to awake and cry. Work your way gently down through the baby's clothing layers.

Student Check-List

- What are the risk factors for developmental dysplasia of the hip?
- What are the signs of heart failure in infancy?
- What diagnosis should be considered in a mucousy baby born to a mother with polyhydramnios? What investigation should be done?
- *The importance of feedback:* students learn and perform better if they receive immediate, authentic and constructive feedback. Without feedback, there is no learning. Three questions for feedback and transfer of learning include: What did you do well in this encounter? What could you do to improve for the next time? What did you learn today that you could use in another clinical situation?

It Happened to me or IGBO (I Got Burnt Once!)

When requesting a baby's blood sugar in an emergency situation, the neonatologist handed a sample to a nearby person without giving the 3 C's of good communication: *Cite* a specific person: "John". Give a *clear* request: "Do a blood glucose on this sample" and *Complete* the communication loop: "Tell me when it's done. "

Each carer, busy in their own tasks of stabilizing the critically ill baby, assumed it was another team member's responsibility to process the blood sugar. It took 30 minutes to appreciate that the sample had not been processed. Fortunately, the subsequent blood glucose was within normal limits and no harm had been done to the baby (a low blood glucose starves the brain of energy and could cause seizures and possible brain injury). The doctor was irritated with himself for this human factor error. However, he resisted the temptation to blame and recalled his mentor referring to mistakes as "instructional friends". He would cite this error as a learning point at the next resuscitation meeting and teach a new mnemonic: ABCDEFG as "Airway, Breathing, Circulation, Don't Ever Forget the Glucose" in sick babies.

There are three classes of people: those who see. Those who see when they are shown. Those who do not see.

Study the science of art and the art of science.

Learn to see and remember that everything is connected to everything else.

Leonardo da Vinci

References

[1] Nishigori H, Masuda K, Kikukawa M, Kawashima A, Yudkowsky R. A model teaching session for the hypothesis-driven physical examination. *Med Teach.* 2011. 33(5);410 -7.

[2] Ganda G, Ibrahim LF, Natchimuthu K, Ryan CA. No more tears: maternal involvement in the neonatal screening examination. *Clin Pediatr* (Phila) 2011. 50(8);753-6.

[3] Fuloria M, Kreiter S. The Newborn Examination: Part I. Emergencies and Common Abnormalities Involving the Skin, Head, Neck, Chest, and Respiratory and Cardiovascular Systems. *Am Fam Physician.* 2002. 1;65(1):61-69.

[4] Fuloria M, Kreiter S The Newborn Examination: Part II. Emergencies and Common Abnormalities Involving the Abdomen, Pelvis, Extremities, Genitalia, and Spine. *Am Fam Physician.* 2002;65(2):265-71.

[5] May M. Neck Masses in children: diagnosis and treatment. *Pediatr Ann* 1976;5:518–35.

In: Learning Clinical Skills
Editors: Bridget Maher and Pat Henn
ISBN: 978-1-62100-409-7

Chapter IX

Examining the Abdomen

David Power and Mark Corrigan

Topic: Small Bowel Obstruction

Clinical Case

A 60 year old female presents to the Emergency Department complaining of generalised abdominal pain, nausea and vomiting. The nausea started two days ago, quickly followed by vomiting. She then noticed that her abdomen was becoming progressively distended and yesterday she started complaining of abdominal pain. She describes this as a peri-umbilical colic and scores it 8/10 at its most severe (0 – no pain, 10 – worst pain ever experienced.) She has been unable to sleep because of the pain and vomiting. She has not eaten in two days and is intolerant of oral fluids.

Her symptoms first occurred while she was at work. She has not eaten anything unusual, has not been abroad in the past year, and has had no contact with other people with similar symptoms. She is passing flatus and it is two days since her last bowel motion. She is very restless and cannot get comfortable. Analgesia (non-steroidal anti-inflammatory) has failed to provide relief from her discomfort. She denies symptoms of dyspepsia, melaena, haematochezia, tenesmus, change of bowel habit or weight loss. There is no family history of colorectal carcinoma, inflammatory bowel disease or coeliac disease.

Past medical history: atrial fibrillation which is rate controlled, dyslipidaemia, hypertension, open appendicectomy for perforated acute appendicitis aged 8 years old.

Medications: warfarin as per INR, atenolol, atorvastatin. She has no known drug allergies and does not take regular over the counter medications or herbal remedies.

Social history: she is a smoker with a forty pack year history and occasionally drinks alcohol. *Review of Systems* is non-contributory.

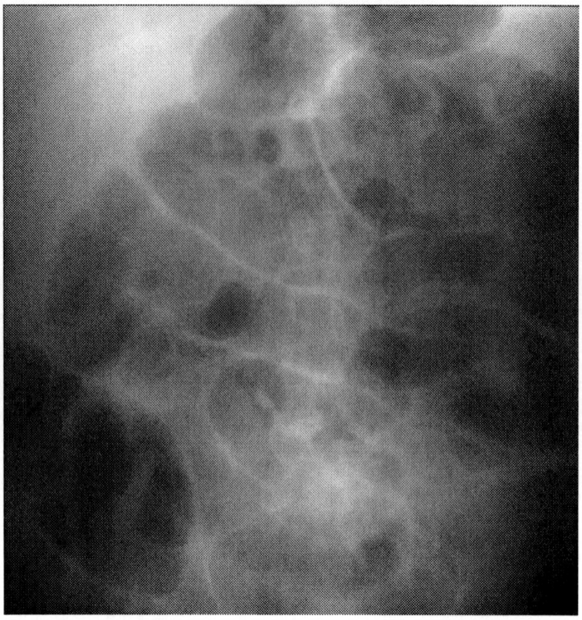

Figure 1. Plain Film Abdomen -Small Bowel Obstruction.

Clinical Examination

The patient is not obviously distressed and is alert and orientated to time, person and place. She is in atrial fibrillation, 85-95 beats per minute and is apyrexial. Her respiratory rate, blood pressure and oxygen saturations are all normal. There are no signs of finger clubbing or pallor of the palmar creases. Skin turgor is increased and her mucous membranes are dry.

Cardiac and respiratory examinations are otherwise normal.

Abdominal examination: Oblique right iliac fossa incision. Distended abdomen. No signs of peritonism. Murphy's sign is negative. No organomegaly. Hernial orifices are clear. Abdomen tympanitic to percussion. No shifting dullness. Tinkling bowel sounds. Rectal examination was normal.

Table 1. Student Dilemma

- Should I do a rectal examination?
- How do I know if it's a small or large bowel obstruction?
- How do I exclude a perforation?
- How do I know that there is no mesenteric ischaemia?

Results: haemoglobin, liver function tests, liver enzyme tests and lactate were all normal. White cell count $13.4x10^9$/L, International Normalised Ratio (INR) 2.3, Sodium 130 mmol/L, Potassium 3.3 mmol/L, Chloride 92 mmol/L, Urea 12.0, Creatinine 95μmol/L. Chest X-Ray normal. Plain film abdomen reveals small bowel obstruction with air fluid levels (Figure 1).

CT Abdomen and Pelvis demonstrated dilated loops of small bowel with a transition point in the distal ileum. No obvious mechanical cause of obstruction identified.
Diagnosis: small bowel obstruction secondary to adhesions.

Discussion

The patient's main complaints are nausea, vomiting, abdominal distension and pain, occurring in that order. In this case, the order in which the symptoms occur is very important. For example, acute appendicitis is classically described as pain followed by nausea and vomiting whereas in gastroenteritis, nausea and vomiting precede the abdominal pain. As is often quoted, 90% of the diagnosis is in the history. To that end, remember to ask all of the relevant questions regarding the nature of the abdominal pain.

The patient reports her abdominal pain as being peri-umbilical and colicky in nature. The site of obstruction may lead to differences in presentation. In proximal small bowel obstruction, vomiting tends to occur earlier, is more profuse and bilious, and leads to dehydration more rapidly. In distal or low small bowel obstruction, vomiting tends to occur later, is less prominent and may be faeculent with pain being a more significant feature. Multiple air-fluid levels are visible on x-ray. The more distal the site of obstruction, the more pronounced the distension. In large bowel obstruction on the other hand, distension occurs late and is marked. Pain is less prominent and dehydration occurs later.

Distension of the small bowel occurs proximal to the site of the obstruction. There are two main causes of this; gas and fluid. In obstruction, there is significant overgrowth of the small bowel flora leading to increased gas production. Proximal to the obstruction, the gastric and small bowel mucosa continue to secrete leading to an accumulation of fluid, whilst gut resorption is impaired. Dehydration and metabolic derangement are the consequence of reduced oral intake, vomiting, impaired gut resorption and sequestration of fluid in the bowel lumen.

Obstipation, or absolute constipation, signifies that the bowel distal to a complete obstruction has been emptied of flatus and faeces. Relative constipation is where only flatus is passed and is present in partial obstruction.

Remember, foregut pain manifests in the upper abdomen, midgut pain in the peri-umbilical region and hindgut pain in the lower abdomen; these are really useful landmarks to know. You just need to remember two points:

- The bile duct opening.
- Two thirds the way along the transverse colon.

Foregut is everything to the bile duct opening; midgut is from the bile duct opening to two-thirds the way along the transverse colon and hindgut is everything past two thirds the way along the transverse colon. Remembering these points makes it easy to remember the blood supply, drainage and innervation of every organ. Foregut is celiac, midgut is superior mesenteric, hindgut is inferior mesenteric. Foregut organs give epigastric pain, midgut organs give periumbilical pain and hindgut organs give suprapubic pain.

The patient's electrolytes are all reduced in the setting of an elevated urea, along with increased skin turgor and dry mucous membranes, indicating that the patient is dehydrated and that she has been obstructed for a prolonged period. A mildly raised white cell count is not uncommon in small bowel obstruction. The patient is warfarinised for her atrial fibrillation and her International Normalised Ratio is 2.3, lying within the desired therapeutic range. Given this patient's cardiac history, serial data should be performed to exclude acute coronary syndrome (unlikely, but this is a serious condition and you don't want to miss it).

Table 2. Describing Pain –SOCRATES

- Site
- Onset
- Character
- Radiation
- Alleviating Factors
- Timing
- Exacerbating Factors
- Severity

The patient's abdomen is obviously distended. The PFA demonstrates dilated loops of small bowel (>3cm diameter) centrally, denoted by valvulae conniventes, with visible air-fluid levels. Thumb-printing denotes the presence of mucosal oedema.

- A CXR does not demonstrate any free air under the diaphragm (a sign of a perforated hollow viscus, but the absence of free air does not exclude a perforation.)
- Abdominal and pelvic Computerized Tomography is an excellent modality for detecting and diagnosing small bowel obstruction. The obstruction can be characterised as partial or complete in nature.
- CT scanning can often also identify the cause of the obstruction and other intra-abdominal pathology such as inflammation, neoplasia and perforation.

Before you begin to examine the patient, take thirty seconds to perform a general inspection.

- Take note of the patient's appearance. Is she distressed, dyspnoac, cyanosed, anaemic or jaundiced?
- What medical paraphernalia are around the bed such as incentive spirometers, sputum cups, dialysis machines, intravenous fluids, nasogastric tube, urinary catheter etc?
- Now examine the patient. Be sure to expose the patient adequately and to carefully inspect, palpate, percuss and auscultate the abdomen. On inspection, you are looking for obvious distension, masses such as herniae and old scars.
- Palpate all areas of the abdomen looking for signs of tenderness/peritonism, possible indicators of ischaemia or perforation. You must examine the hernial orifices as

herniae are the second most frequent cause of small bowel obstruction after adhesions.

- Auscultate for bowel sounds. These may be absent in paralytic ileus or tinkling in mechanical obstruction.
- Percuss the abdomen listening for hyper-resonance (occurs in the presence of dilated loops of bowel).
- A rectal examination is mandatory: therefore position the patient in the left lateral position with their hips and knees flexed. You are looking for the presence of a rectal mass or impacted faeces.

It is important to consider the various causes of small bowel obstruction. These can be considered in terms of intra-luminal, bowel wall and extra-luminal causes

Table 3. Causes of Small Bowel Obstruction

- Intra-luminal: food bolus, gallstone ileus, foreign bodies, meconium ileus
- Bowel wall: inflammation (Crohn's disease), neoplasia, ischaemia, stricture, congenital atresia
- Extra-luminal: herniae, adhesions, volvulus, intussusception, tumours

Table 4. Intestinal Obstruction

Symptoms

- Colicky central abdominal pain
- Absolute constipation
- Nausea, vomiting

Signs

- Abdominal distention
- Visible peristalsis
- Percussion - hyper-resonant
- Auscultation – high, pitched, tinkling bowel sounds
- Check for herniae, masses, scars

Small bowel obstruction can also be described as mechanical or adynamic in nature. In mechanical obstruction, the bowel peristalses against a mechanical obstruction. In adynamic obstruction, peristalsis may be present (Ogilvie's syndrome) or absent (paralytic ileus).

Strangulation occurs when the blood supply to the small bowel is impaired. This results in increased capillary pressure and therefore increased fluid shifts. When the arterial supply is compromised, this results in mesenteric ischaemia, infarction and perforation. External herniae tend to involve less bowel than internal herniae and consequently have a better outcome. The greater the amount of involved bowel - the more significant the blood loss and fluid shift - the more severe the degree of shock and the worse the prognosis.

Lab-Spot

- In early small bowel obstruction there may be no abnormalities in the blood results.
- As dehydration progresses, sodium, potassium and chloride may decrease while urea and creatinine may rise (depending on severity).
- The white cell count may rise and is associated with strangulation and a worse prognosis.
- A mild amylasaemia can be observed, released from small bowel mucosa
- An elevated lactate may be indicative of bowel ischaemia, but lactate can be raised in sepsis, shock, diabetic ketoacidosis, ethanol ingestion etc.

Pearls

- Note the order in which the symptoms arise – pain and then nausea and vomiting in acute appendicitis versus nausea and vomiting followed by pain in other conditions such as gastroenteritis.
- Remember the two embryological points: the bile duct opening and two-thirds the way along the transverse colon.
- Position the patient correctly – head on one pillow, arms lying flat by sides and legs uncrossed.
- Expose the patient adequately so as not to miss any scars/masses.
- Take note of any medical paraphernalia around the bedside.
- Take time to perform a general inspection – you will glean much valuable information.
- On inspection, look carefully for old laparoscopic scars as these are easily missed.
- Look at the patient's face while palpating the abdomen.
- Carefully examine the hernial orifices both lying and standing.
- No abdominal examination is complete without examining the rectum and the scrotum in males.
- When performing a rectal examination, do not miss the opportunity to check for faecal occult blood.
- Apply "SOCRATES" when taking a history of abdominal pain.
- Know the differential diagnoses of abdominal pain and bowel obstruction.

Pitfalls

- Introduce yourself at the beginning.
- Start palpating the abdomen at the site furthest from any pain.
- Examine the hernial orifices.
- Do not be afraid to correctly position the patient if they are not already in the correct position – this may be a deliberate ploy by the examiners.

- Always inspect the back – this is often forgotten and is also an important part of the abdominal examination.

Tips for the OSCE

- Arrive early for your examination
- Introduce yourself to each patient, be courteous, smile, and thank the patient at the end of the examination
- Wash your hands before and after examining each patient
- Clean your stethoscope between patients
- Be confident and definite in what you say
- Include relevant positive and negative findings

Student Check List

- What is a hernia?
- How do I tell the difference between a direct and indirect inguinal hernia?
- What are the foregut, midgut and hindgut?
- What's the difference between small and large bowel obstruction?
- What are the aetiologies of small bowel obstruction?
- What are the commonest herniae in men and women?

Table 5. Abdominal pain-Visceral and Somatic

Visceral -Pain from hollow viscera –'colic'

- Crampy/paroxysmal
- Often poorly localised
- Related to peristalsis

Somatic -Pain from peritonal irritation

- Steady/constant
- Often well localised
- Not related to peristalsis
- Patient often lies still with knees up

It Happened to me

A 76 year old man with a distended abdomen was seen by the doctor on-call. The patient had pain radiating out his back, no bowel motion for three days and dehydration with a tachycardia and hypotension. The doctor had suspected a bowel obstruction as the PFA demonstrated some dilated loops of bowel and had ordered a CT scan. The patient died in X-ray from a ruptured aortic aneurysm.

1. Always, always beware the elderly patient with back pain. Suspect the worst and you'll be wrong a lot, but one day you'll be right.
2. Never send a patient to the x-ray department who is haemodynamically unstable. If a patient is that unwell, he needs to be near the resuscitation room and the operating theatre. The x-ray department is not the place for resuscitation.
3. The absence of a bowel motion for three days was a red herring which was seized upon by the doctor as it neatly explained what he had decided was the diagnosis.

In the words of William Osler, "*you can't diagnose what you haven't thought of.*" Throughout your career, always consider the common diagnosis, and the most serious diagnosis.

In: Learning Clinical Skills
Editors: Bridget Maher and Pat Henn
ISBN: 978-1-62100-409-7

Chapter X

The Diabetic Foot: Pearls, Pitfalls and Tips for the OSCE

Antoinette Tuthill

Clinical Case

A 67-year old man presented to the Accident and Emergency Department complaining of redness and swelling of his right forefoot. His foot was not painful and he had only become aware of the swelling after it was pointed out to him by his daughter. Although he had been advised to always wear a hard-soled shoe/ sandal/slipper on his feet, he frequently forgot to do this, to and liked to walk barefoot around the house instead.

He has a past history of type 2 diabetes for 15 years and has had laser therapy for retinopathy; he has had persistent microalbuminuria for the last five years and ceased smoking two years prior to presentation. His history was also significant for hypertension, hyperlipidaemia, obesity and previous stent insertion to his right coronary artery.

Medications on presentation included a sulphonylurea, metformin, aspirin and a statin. His last HbA_{1c} was 8.9% (74 mmol/mol) reflecting glucose levels regularly in double figures.

Clinical Examination: BP 145/88 mmHg, apyrexial, heart rate 96 regular, BMI 34 kg/m^2 with a central distribution of body fat.

Examination of the cardiovascular system revealed a right carotid bruit and decreased, but palpable, peripheral pulses bilaterally at the level of the popliteal artery. The right dorsalis pedis and posterior tibial pulses were barely palpable, although they could be appreciated using Doppler waveform analysis. Capillary refill time was prolonged in the right great toe.
Respiratory and abdominal examinations were within normal limits.

Lower Limbs: There was marked erythema and swelling of the right forefoot in comparison with the left forefoot and the patient was wearing a dressing on the plantar surface of his forefoot which he reported that his public health nurse had applied one week previously. Removal of the dressing revealed a foul-smelling green discharge from a deep ulcer and surrounding erythema. Once the discharge was cleared, bone appeared to be visible in the wound bed.

He had absent monofilament perception on both feet and loss of proprioception to the level of the ankle joints bilaterally. Using a tuning fork, he demonstrated absent vibration perception to the level of the tibial tuberosity on the right, and to the level of the medial malleolus on the left. Knee and ankle reflexes were present bilaterally and were symmetrical.

Diagnosis: Mixed neuropathic and ischaemic ulcer with possible underlying osteomyelitis.

Student Dilemma

- How do I tell if an ulcer is ischaemic or neuropathic in origin?
- What are the clues from the history that the patient was at risk of both microvascular and macrovascular disease?
- Should I comment on footwear?
- What was the likely infective organism responsible for the green discharge from the wound?
- What would make you suspect that the patient had an underlying osteomyelitis?
- How do I use a monofilament?
- When do I refer for vascular assessment?

Discussion

The patient has a history of both macrovascular (history of previous coronary artery stent insertion and detectable carotid bruit on examination) and microvascular disease (history of persistent microalbuminuria and requirement for laser treatment of eye disease). His elevated blood pressure and the presence of central obesity are two modifiable risk factors that can be addressed by encouraging lifestyle change (diet and exercise) in addition to intensification of therapy to achieve blood pressure control. He also gives a history of smoking until two years prior to presentation and his most recent HbA_{1c} of 8.9% (74 mmol/mol) suggests that his glucose control is not satisfactory (HbA_{1c} provides a measure of average levels of glucose over the preceding 2-3 months. It reflects the degree to which the patient's haemoglobin has been glycosylated over that time interval). Options to improve glycaemic control in a patient on metformin and a sulphonylurea include lifestyle change, dose titration, addition of a third oral agent (such as a thiazolidinedione or a dipeptidyl peptidase-4 inhibitor), consideration of either basal insulin initiation (risks of hypoglycaemia and weight gain) or commencement of a glucagon-like peptide-1 analogue/agonist (aids weight loss in addition to improving glycaemic control).

Improper or poorly fitting shoes are major contributors to foot ulceration in patients with diabetes. All patients with diabetes need to pay special attention to the fit and style of their shoes and should avoid pointed-toe shoes or high heels. Evaluation of the feet of patients with diabetes for risk of ulceration involves inspecting for deformities and skin changes, assessment of circulatory status and assessment for neuropathy (Figures 1,2,3). Prevention of foot problems requires patient education, podiatry, regular foot inspection and assessment and advice regarding appropriate footwear (Figure 4).

The gentleman in this case had previously received footcare advice regarding the need to always wear hard-soled footwear and to examine his feet regularly either using a mirror or by asking a family member to inspect them daily, but he appears to have been poorly compliant with this advice. Re-education of the patient and family members to avoid further preventable complications developing as a result of diabetes is a key part of management. The absence of pain in his foot, in addition to the clinical findings on examination, suggests the presence of neuropathy which would have contributed to his increased risk of sustaining an injury.

The green, malodourous discharge from the ulcer would prompt suspicion of infection with pseudomonas. Culture of the discharge may help guide the choice of appropriate antibiotics. Osteomyelitis must always be considered in an ulcer which appears to probe to bone. Measurement of ESR, CRP and a foot X-ray would be appropriate first-line investigations for osteomyelitis; occasionally an isotope bone scan or MRI is useful for evaluation if there is a high clinical suspicion of osteomyelitis but there is no evidence of bone destruction on plain films.

Charcot's osteoarthropathy needs to be considered in patients with evidence of peripheral and/or autonomic neuropathy and a good blood supply to the lower limb (Figure 2). Increased blood flow due to sympathethic nerve loss can cause an increase in osteoclast activity and bone turnover making the bones of the foot more susceptible to damage. Even minor trauma can therefore result in destructive changes in this susceptible bone. The most common sites affected are the tarsal-metatarsal region or the metatarsophalangeal joints. Initially, Charcot's osteoarthropathy causes a warm swollen foot which may be indistinguishable from cellulitis or gout. Cellulitis is more likely in the presence of an ulcer which may show typical signs of infection. Infection and Charcot's arthropathy can sometimes be present concurrently in the same foot. If in doubt, treat for both. Immobilisation and/or bisphosphonates may help to prevent development of the bone destruction and deformity associated with this condition.

A carotid ultrasound should be performed to evaluate the degree of stenosis present given that the patient has multiple risk factors for a cerebrovascular event.

Table 1. Features used to describe an ulcer

- Site
- Size
- Appearance of ulcer and surrounding tissues
- Discharge
- Associated swelling
- Tenderness
- Smell
- Depth and dimensions (determined by probing)

Table 2.Features that help differentiate betweeen Ischaemic and Neuropathic ulcers[*]

	Ischaemic	Neuropathic
Temperature	Normal or cool	Warm
Pulses	Absent	Present
Pain	Sometimes severe	None
Site	Lateral borders of feet (areas susceptible to friction / shear)	Under toes and metatarsal heads (areas susceptible to high pressure)
Depth	Shallow	Deep
Callus	Minimal	Often heavy callus

Right lower extremity angiography in conjunction with vascular surgery referral should be performed to evaluate whether the patient has a significant stenosis in the arteries to his right leg which would be amenable to dilatation (angioplasty +/- stenting) or bypass surgery in order to facilitate healing of the forefoot ulcer.

Mixed ischaemic/neuropathic ulcers are often present in patients with diabetes.

Pitfalls

- In a patient with diabetes, it is important to always examine the lower limbs in detail, removing all dressings and looking beneath, even if the patient does not complain of lower extremity pain. You may miss a previous amputation site, or the source of the patient's underlying sepsis.
- Even shallow-appearing ulcers in a patient with diabetes must be appropriately evaluated for possible underlying osteomyelitis.
- Infection is the commonest complication of diabetes.

Pearls

- Patients with diabetes who have absent monofilament perception on the feet are at increased risk of foot ulceration and must receive appropriate footcare advice and examination on a regular basis (at least annually); they need to be advised to avoid walking barefoot (including on hot sand while on holiday – risk of sustaining burns), and to self-examine their feet daily. Regular moisturiser will also help to reduce the risk of dry skin which can crack, leading to an increased risk of ulceration.
- A painless ulcer should raise the suspicion of underlying neuropathy.
- Mixed ischaemic/neuropathic ulcers are common in patients with diabetes.
- Vascular examination of the lower limbs is best performed by starting proximally (groin) and proceeding distally; neurological examination of the lower limbs in a patient with diabetes is best performed by starting at the periphery and working proximally to locate the level of the neuropathy.
- Always compare one limb with the other.

- Urinalysis is an easy bedside/clinic test to evaluate for microvascular disease in diabetes; a patient with diabetes who demonstrates the presence of microvascular disease in one area is at much higher risk of microvascular disease in other areas.
- Many diabetic patients have medial arterial calcification, giving an artificially elevated systolic pressure in the feet even in the presence of ischaemia; this may result in an ankle brachial pressure index (ABPI) of > 1 (the ratio of ankle systolic pressure to brachial systolic pressure). It is then necessary to use other methods to assess flow in the arteries of the foot, such as examining the pattern of Doppler arterial waveform or measuring transcutaneous oxygen tension ($TcPO_2$), a measurement of oxygen perfusion of the skin.
- A low risk foot patient has normal foot pulses, normal vibration (128Hz tuning fork) and sensation to 10g monofilament, no history of foot ulceration, no significant foot deformity and no visual impairment.

Tips for the OSCE

Examination of the feet in a patient with diabetes should involve:

- Inspection of the skin, nails and foot structure (for deformity e.g. hallux valgus, high arch foot, claw toe or Charcot foot) (figures 1, 2).
- Sensory testing using a 10g monofilament and vibration perception testing (figure 3).
- Palpation of foot pulses (dorsalis pedis and posterior tibial).
- Examination of footwear (figure 4).

In the untreated patient with Charcot's osteoarthropathy, two classic midfoot deformities are seen:

- A 'rocker bottom' deformity due to displacement and subluxation of the tarsus downwards.
- Medial convexity due to displacement of the talonavicular joint or tarsometatarsal dislocation.

Sensory Assessment of the Foot in Diabetes

Cutaneous Pressure Assessment (10g monofilament) delivers a 10-gram force when properly applied. Research has shown that a person who can feel the 10-gram filament in the selected sites is at reduced risk for developing ulcers.

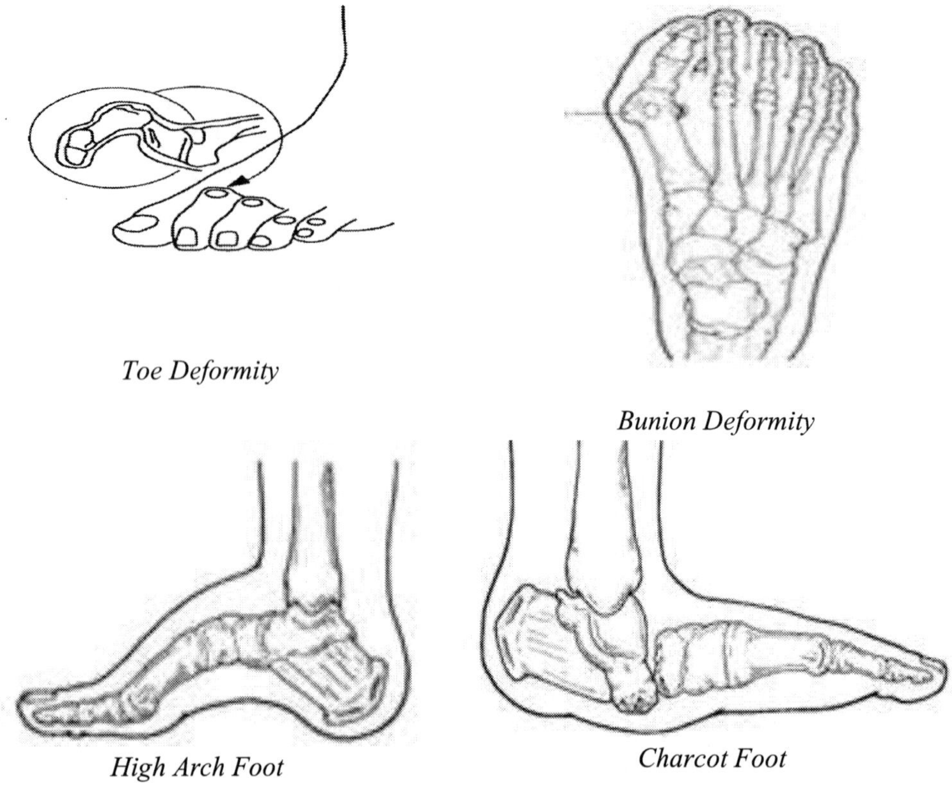

Figure 1. Structural Foot Deformity.

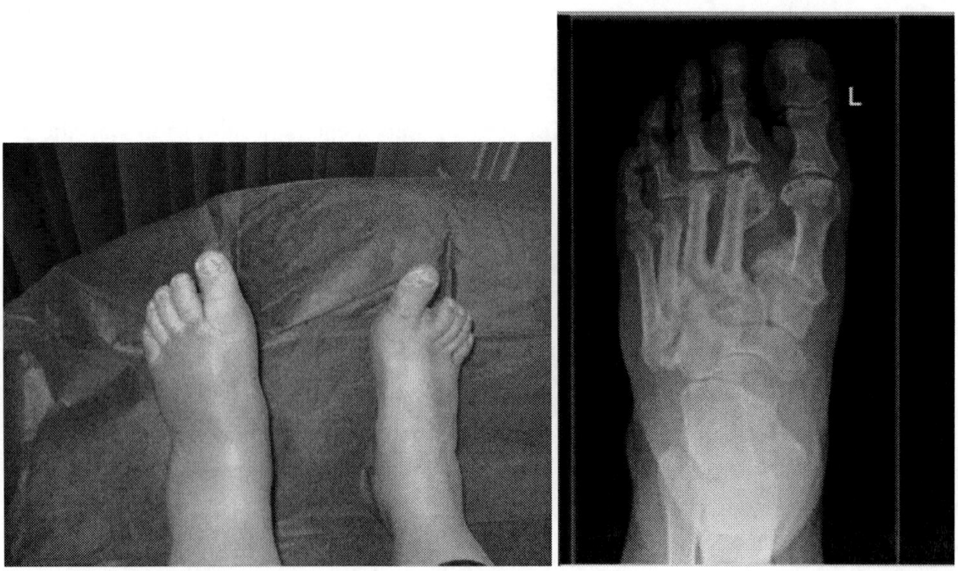

Figure 2. A Charcot foot.

- The sensory exam should be done in a quiet and relaxed setting. The patient must not watch while the examiner applies the filament.
- Test the monofilament on the patient's hand so he/she knows what to anticipate.
- The four sites to be tested are indicated below.
- Apply the monofilament perpendicular to the skin's surface (A)
- Apply sufficient force to cause the filament to bend or buckle (B)
- The total duration of the approach, skin contact, and departure of the filament should be approximately 1-1.5 seconds.
- Apply the filament along the perimeter and NOT ON an ulcer site, callus, scar or necrotic tissue. Do not allow the filament to slide across the skin or make repetitive contact at the test site.
- Press the filament to the skin such that it buckles at one of two times as you say "time one" or "time two." Have patients identify at which time they were touched. Randomise the sequence of applying the filament throughout the examination.

If the patient cannot feel the filament at any of the tested areas, then protective foot sensation is lost, indicating susceptibility to ulceration.

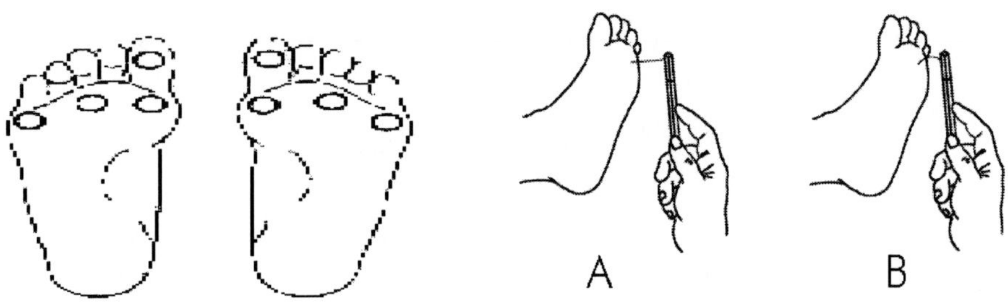

Figure 3. Sensory Assessment of the foot in Diabetes.

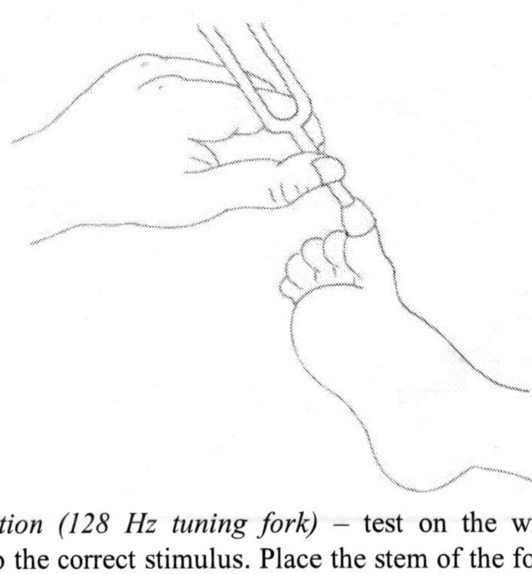

C *Vibration Testing*

Vibration Perception (128 Hz tuning fork) – test on the wrist first to ensure that the patient is responding to the correct stimulus. Place the stem of the fork over the tip of the big toe (figure C) and ask the patient to tell you if they feel vibration. Record the result as absent, reduced or present depending on the patient's response.

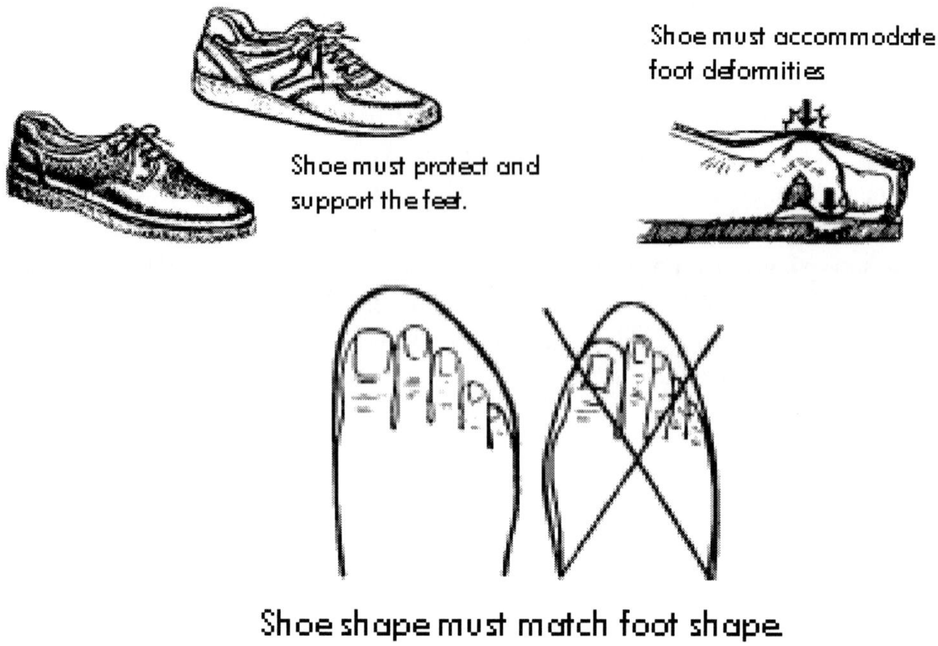

Figure 4. Footwear Assessment.

Student Checklist

- What features help to differentiate between ischaemic and neuropathic feet?
- What are the essential components of a foot examination in a patient with diabetes?
- What type of structural foot deformities may be present?
- What are the consequences of microvascular disease in patients with diabetes?
- How do you use a monofilament to test for neuropathy?

It Happened to me

A 42-year old lady with a three month history of palpitations, increased anxiety and insomnia recently presented to the Accident and Emergency Department. Three weeks prior to admission, she had been diagnosed with Graves' disease (antibody-mediated thyrotoxicosis) and was started on anti-thyroid drugs. In the two weeks immediately preceding presentation, she described fevers, recurrent vomiting and left shoulder tip pain. Recorded observations in the Accident and Emergency Department showed her to be pyrexial, tachycardic and hypotensive; examination revealed a coarse tremor, and thyroid function tests revealed persistent thyrotoxicosis.

She was referred to the endocrinology service with a provisional diagnosis of thyroid storm.

Thyroid storm is a rare, life-threatening condition (30-50% mortality) which can occur in an individual with thyrotoxicosis – it often manifests with persistent pyrexia, tachycardia, altered mental status, nausea and vomiting, abnormal liver function tests and cardiovascular instability.

Further review of this lady revealed her to have a lower respiratory chest infection with her symptoms being consistent with a systemic inflammatory response. She responded well to a course of antibiotic therapy. *Common things are common.*

The part can never be well unless the whole is well.

Plato

References

Edmonds M.E., Foster A.V.M., Sanders L.J. (2004). *A Practical Manual of Diabetic Footcare*. Oxford: Blackwell Publishing.

Watkins P.J., Amiel S.A., Howell S.L. and Turner E. (2004). *Diabetes and its Management* (Sixth Edition). London: Blackwell Publishing.

In: Learning Clinical Skills
Editors: Bridget Maher and Pat Henn
ISBN: 978-1-62100-409-7

Chapter XI

Shock and Collapse in the Emergency Department

Stephen Cusack

Topic: Shock

Clinical Case

A 71 year old female arrives by ambulance to the Emergency Department at around 11a.m. Her husband had become alarmed when she was unable to sit up in bed without feeling extremely dizzy and he was also concerned that she seemed drowsy.

The patient complained of feeling weak and cold. She said that her symptoms commenced the previous evening when she had felt suddenly cold and weak. She then vomited on about three occasions. She was not certain what the vomitus contained but there may have been frank blood and it may have been coffee coloured but she was not sure. She had not had any bowel movements. She had no pain. A systems review was otherwise unremarkable.

Past medical history: The patient has a long history of dyspepsia and her symptoms have been under control for years with omeprazole. She has Rheumatoid Arthritis for 15 years and takes methotrexate. She has recently commenced a course of prednisone for a 'flare up' of arthritic symptoms. The patient has been taking an SSRI for depression for many years. She was treated for urinary tract infections on two or three occasions in the last two years by her family doctor. She is taking a calcium channel blocker for hypertension.

Clinical Examination: The patient is pale and subdued (almost to the point of drifting to sleep during conversation) but fully oriented. She is cool to touch. Capillary refill time is prolonged (>2 seconds), pulse 94/minute and regular, respiratory rate 22/minute, and blood pressure is 70 mmHg systolic. Oxygen saturations are 94% on room air, improving to 97% on high flow oxygen.

Examination of the respiratory and cardiovascular systems and abdominal examination are all unremarkable.

Initial test results: WCC is 19x $10^3/\mu L$ (upper limit 11), Haemoglobin is 10.5g/dl (lower limit 12.5) and HCT is 0.29. Venous biochemistry is normal. Temperature is 35.5C. A Chest X-ray is normal and urine is initially not available. An ECG is unremarkable with no diagnostic changes. Blood sugar is 8.6 mmol/lt.

Table 1. Student Dilemma

- Is the patient in shock?
- What is the cause?
- What further information can help?
- What must be done?

Discussion

Shock is a condition where there is failure to perfuse vital organs and tissues with oxygenated blood and nutrients. Clinically this is recognised where there is alteration in consciousness, poor peripheral perfusion, tachypnoea, and hypotension (systolic BP< 90mmHg) with or without a tachycardia (which is influenced by age, fitness, medications and is also dependent on cardiac function).

Clinically this patient is in shock. The end organ evidence is primarily seen in relation to her brain perfusion (altered level of consciousness), cool skin and peripheral perfusion (capillary refill >2 seconds), and cardiovascular function (hypotension). It is particularly important to note that patients do not have altered mental status without good reason. It is not normal for people to be drowsy, sleepy or confused, yet it is surprising how frequently this is passed over as unremarkable, especially by young doctors and students who think that anyone over 45 has probably slowed down mentally to the point of permanent drowsiness!

Some important clues in this patient's presentation are her drug history (which include two immunosuppressants -methotrexate and steroids) and a history of previous urinary sepsis. An elevated WCC is helpful in pointing towards sepsis in this case. However, it is important to know that the WCC may be normal or low in septic patients and to remember that steroids can cause leucocytosis, although 19 is probably a little high for simple steroid induced leucocytosis.

The ECG shows no acute changes or signs of ischaemia and the patient has no history of chest pain or ischaemic heart disease. This is helpful. However, painless acute myocardial infarction is not uncommon and the first ECG will be normal in up to 30% of patients presenting to the Emergency Department with acute myocardial infarction. Cardiac enzymes may help but highly sensitive troponin will be elevated in many acute situations including severe sepsis and gastrointestinal haemorrhage.

The patient also gives a possible history of haematemesis and there is a background of upper gastrointestinal symptoms treated with a proton pump inhibitor which could possibly suggest peptic ulcer disease as the underlying problem. Initial haemoglobin is 10.5g/dl and HCT is slightly below normal so haemorrhage is still a possibility.

Table 2. Classification of Shock

Hypovolaemic

- Blood loss- trauma, GI bleed, ectopic pregnancy, abdominal aortic aneurysm
- Fluid loss (3rd Spacing)- GI loss (vomiting/diarrhoea), burns, sepsis, pancreatitis

Cardiogenic

- Primary- MI, arrythmia, myocarditis
- Secondary- tamponade, PE, tension pneumothorax

Septic

- Immunocompromise- drugs, malignancy, diabetes
- Obvious site- chest, urinary, abdomen, skin

Other: anaphylactic, neurogenic, endocrine-DM, Addison's), poisoning (usually drugs)

Table 3. SIRS Criteria

- Temperature >38C or <36C
- RR >20/min or pCO2 <4.16kPa
- Heart rate > 90/min
- WCC < 4 or >12
- The presence of 2 or more of the above PLUS EITHER
- Systolic BP < 90mmHg or MAP<65mmHg
- OR Lactate =/> 4mmol/lt

The patient's serum venous biochemistry and blood glucose and drug and allergy history mean that anaphylaxis, endocrine abnormality, and poisoning are not really a significant concern. There are no features to suggest that neurogenic shock is part of the differential diagnosis.

The patient's clinical presentation and initial findings suggest that haemorrhagic or septic shock are the first major considerations. To further assist in diagnosing septic shock, it is important to be aware of the Systemic Inflammatory Response Syndrome (SIRS) and the criteria for diagnosing this response.

Clinically, this patient fulfils the SIRS criteria for severe sepsis. An Arterial Blood Gas (ABG) is a useful additional investigation in this situation and it is important to obtain a urine sample at the earliest opportunity. This will require placing a urinary catheter.

Results of an ABG analysis show a pCO2 of 4 and a lactate of 4.6. Meanwhile, a urine sample reveals a WCC on microscopy of over 500.

This patient has severe sepsis. This is a common presenting emergency. It is estimated that over 1,400 people die every day in the world from sepsis and that around 37,000 people die each year in the UK. Early recognition and intervention are important. Management involves the ABC approach with reservation of blood cultures and early administration (within 1 hour of presentation) of an appropriate antibiotic. The Survive Sepsis campaign in the UK asserts that if treatment for sepsis is commenced within one hour of arrival in the Emergency Department, then mortality can be reduced significantly. To this end, the campaign advocates adopting use of the “Sepsis Six”. These represent six straightforward actions that can be taken by any health professional before instigation of specialist therapy. Quite simply the “Sepsis Six” are:

1. Give high flow oxygen (via non-rebreather mask)
2. Take blood cultures
3. Give IV antibiotics
4. Start IV fluid resuscitation (crystalloid)
5. Check haemoglobin and lactate
6. Monitor accurate hourly urine output (may require catheter)

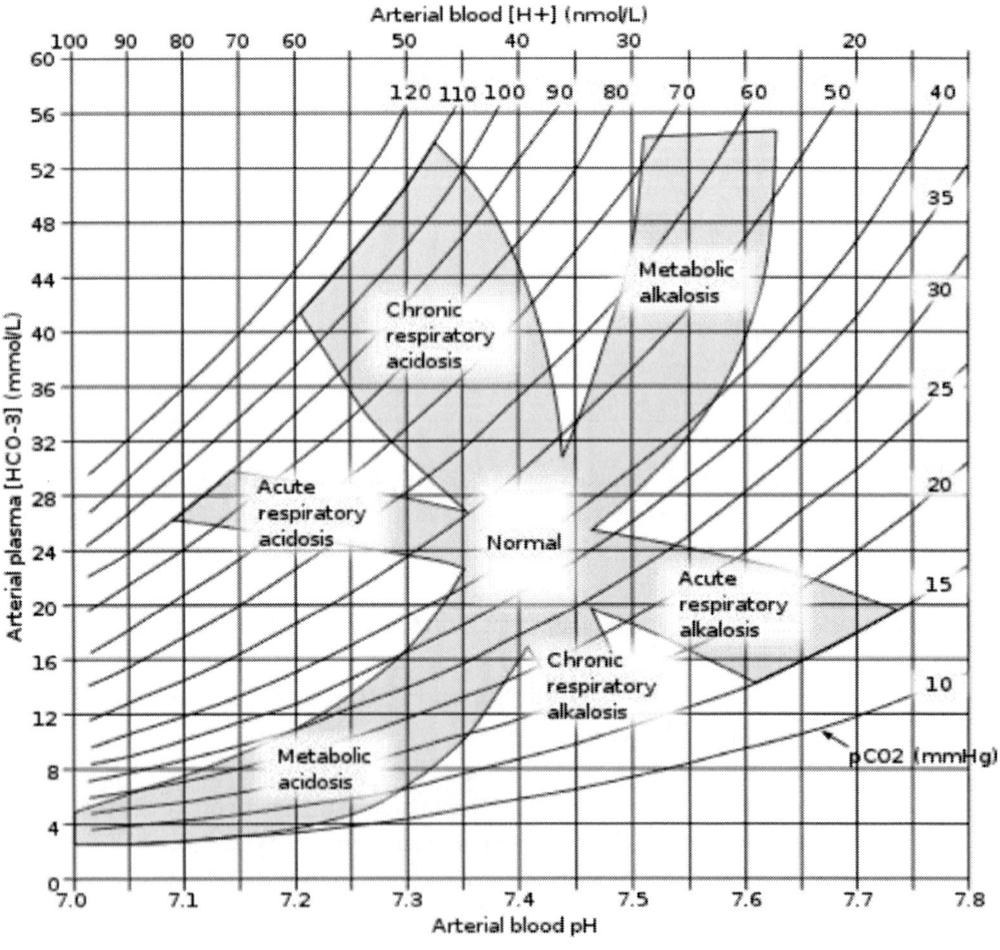

Figure 1. Acid Base Nomogram.

Collapse

The word 'collapse' is often used loosely by lay and professional people to describe a sudden event affecting an individual. A dictionary definition includes 1. 'To fall down or cave in suddenly', 2. 'To fail completely', 3.'To break down or fall down from lack of strength', 4.'A sudden failure or breakdown' (Collins English Dictionary).

Syncope, on the other hand, is a sudden loss of consciousness with subsequent complete recovery. Syncope, therefore, has at its heart a loss of consciousness while 'collapse' may not in fact involve a loss of consciousness. The patient described in the clinical scenario above has had a collapse. She did not have a syncope and at no point was there a suggestion that she was going to make a complete and unassisted recovery. Once down, the collapsed patient tends to stay down, unless there is active intervention. By definition, the syncopal patient makes an initial complete recovery, and the challenge is to determine the underlying cause of the syncopal episode.

Classic syncope is the simple faint. It is neurally mediated and not uncommon. It usually has a prodrome involving feeling hot or nauseated and may be associated with situations involving prolonged standing or psychogenic triggers such as seeing blood and so forth. It can be associated with prolonged fasting (or sometimes overindulgence) and alcohol. If the fainter cannot become supine, they may start to develop convulsive-like twitching (convulsive syncope). It is therefore critical to establish exactly what happened and what was seen by witnesses.

The question can often arise as to whether the patient had a seizure or a faint. Seizures usually involve generalised tonic-clonic movement, incontinence and tongue biting. Patients usually have a period of post convulsive drowsiness or diminished consciousness.

Syncope is never an exertionally related phenomenon. If associated with exertion, then an underlying cardiac abnormality is possible. Some cardiac abnormalities are associated with sudden collapse (HOCM, Stokes-Adams attacks, sudden arrhythmias) so factors such as age, a history of palpitations, past medical history, family history, and physical examination findings are important.

Syncope may also be seen in the context of blood loss (GI bleeds), ectopic pregnancy, large vessel dissections (Aorta, carotids), PE, or following intracranial catastrophe (subarachnoid haemorrhage).Any patient experiencing syncope should have a full history and proper physical evaluation. If appropriate, a rectal examination may help in detecting GI bleeding. Blood glucose should be measured and an ECG is invaluable.

Table 4. Tips for the OSCE

- Remember your PPE (or at least say you'd use them!)
- Adopt the ABC approach
- Know what normal vital signs are
- Have a method to interpret the ECG
- Understand the ABG

It Happened to me

I was on duty as the Emergency Medicine Registrar in a large Department in Scotland which was associated with an eminent medical school. It was about 11.30pm. An ambulance crew arrived with a man on a stretcher. They weren't sure what they wanted to do with the patient. They had picked the patient up in response to a call to a very respectable neighbourhood. The patient had last been seen by his wife at about 10pm when he had gone in to the study with his customary nocturnal glass of whisky (Scotch Malt, naturally). Subsequently, his wife heard shouting and discovered her husband in an agitated state when she went to the study. The Paramedics found the patient sitting on a chair mumbling and the man appeared to have vomited. The smell of drink was overwhelming.

When I initially approached the crew, my first reaction was to the overpowering smell of alcohol. The patient was responding to shouting his name loudly. The impression was that he was very drunk indeed. When I shouted the name for a second time, it struck me that it had a familiar ring. I suddenly realised that I was shouting the name of the Professor of Medicine! This made me stop, and reconsider my first impressions. We moved the patient into the resuscitation room. It wasn't long before it became difficult to move in the room because of consultants crowding in from all directions and most specialties. The patient died a few hours later. He had suffered a massive subarachnoid haemorrhage.

Moral: Not everyone who smells of drink is intoxicated to the point of semi-consciousness and subarachnoid haemorrhage is a common and deadly condition.

Live neither in the past nor in the future, but let each day absorb all your interest, energy and enthusiasm. The best preparation for tomorrow is to live today superbly well.

Sir William Osler

Further Reading

Collins Softback English Dictionary, 3rd Ed. Glasgow: HarperCollins Publishers; 1991.

Dellinger RP, Levy MM, Carlet JM, et. al: Surviving Sepsis Campaign: International guidelines for management of severe sepsis and septic shock: 2008 [published correction appears in *Crit Care Med* 2008; 36:1394-1396]. *Crit Care Med* 2008; 36:296-327.

National Institute for Health and Clinical Excellence, Guideline Development Group. Transient Loss of Consciousness ('Blackouts') Management in Adults and Young People.2010[2011July3] http://www.nice.org.uk/nicemedia/live/13111/50452/50452.pdf

Nutbeam, T. *Survive Sepsis Website.* 2010 [2011 July 3]. Available from: http://www. survivesepsis.org/

O'Sullivan, I. Severe Sepsis. 2008 [2011 July 3]. Available from: http://www. handbook. muh.ie/Infections/severe_sepsis.

Wyatt, JP, Illingworth, RN, Graham, CA, Clancy, MJ, Robertson, CE, *Oxford Handbook of Emergency Medicine,* 3rd Edition. Oxford: Oxford University Press; 2006.

In: Learning Clinical Skills
Editors: Bridget Maher and Pat Henn
ISBN: 978-1-62100-409-7

Chapter XII

D is for Dyspnoea

John Hinchion

Clinical Case

A 74 year old lady attended her doctor. She was accompanied by her family who were concerned that she was getting short of breath. The patient says that she is just getting old and that they are worrying unnecessarily. The breathlessness has been present for the past 18 months and is progressive. Initially the patient was able to walk one mile comfortably on flat ground but now she is breathless after approximately 100 metres or less. On direct questioning, she gives a long history of avoiding hills while walking and gets palpitations and has to 'stop for a few seconds' when she reaches the top of her stairs at home. She smoked 30 years ago for 5 years and never worked in a job that affected her breathing or health. The patient's legs are mildly swollen at night which she ascribes to longstanding varicose veins which she developed during pregnancy many years ago. She is taking levo-thyroxine for hypothyroidism. She has been taking a calcium channel blocker for hypertension for the past 15 years. The patient does not volunteer a history of chest pain, but on further questioning, complains of heaviness in her chest which occurs when she rushes somewhere or gets excited/upset. Occasionally she feels faint if she gets up suddenly. No history of orthopnoea or paroxysmal nocturnal dyspnoea. The family history is positive for coronary artery disease. The patient is a widow and lives alone. Review of other systems is non-contributory. Clinical examination is remarkable for evidence of dyspnoea on mobilisation to the examination couch. Heart rate regular, 70bpm. Blood pressure 115/90, cool peripheries. No clinical evidence of anaemia. The jugular venous pulse is visible 2cm above the sternal notch with the patient examined at a 45 degree angle. There is no evidence of a right ventricular heave, however, the apex beat is very easily felt in the 5th intercostal space 2cm lateral to the mid-clavicular line. There is an ejection systolic murmur at the base of the heart which is best heard in the second right intercostal space adjacent to the sternum. It radiates to both carotids. There is a faint diastolic murmur at the lower left sternal border which is difficult to hear.

Examination of the respiratory system is unremarkable. In particular, there is no evidence of any crepitations at lung bases. There is no evidence of an enlarged liver or sacral oedema. Examination of the lower limbs reveals peripheral oedema to the lower third of the leg and varicose veins are visible bilaterally.

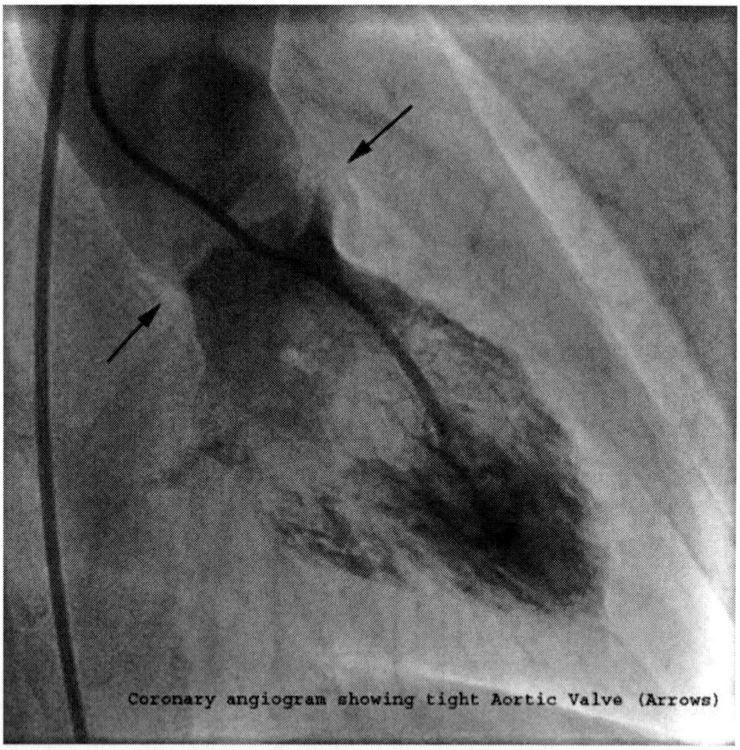

Figure 1. Location of stenotic aortic valve in an angiographic study
(Photograph courtesy of Mr Saleem Jahangeer, Department of Cardio-Thoracic Surgery, Cork University Hospital, Cork).

The patient underwent further investigations and had echocardiography and coronary angiography. A diagnosis of severe aortic stenosis and mild aortic incompetence was established.

Student Dilemma

- Is dyspnoea respiratory or cardiac in origin?
- How do I interpret or quantify dyspnoea?
- How do I more easily hear a faint murmur?
- Does angina mean the patient has chest pain?
- Is observation relevant in the examination of a patient with cardiac disease?

Discussion

Dyspnoea, angina and syncope are the primary symptoms of aortic stenosis.
Dyspnoea is a common symptom. It is broadly either respiratory or cardiac in origin. A patient may describe the symptom of dyspnoea as fatigue. It is very important, however, to clearly establish the symptom as that of dyspnoea. The symptom of fatigue is much less specific and has a multiplicity of causes. In this particular case, the patient may be either hypo or hyperthyroid if the dose of L-Thyroxine is inappropriate. This could cause fatigue. It is also important to appreciate that thyroid pathophysiology is a cause of cardiac symptoms e.g. palpitations and heart failure.

The symptom of dyspnoea may also be associated with coronary ischaemia. A patient may have angina equivalent dyspnoea whereby the typical symptom of anginal discomfort is replaced by the symptom of dyspnoea due to left ventricular ischaemic dysfunction on exercise with concomitant pulmonary venous congestion.

In relation to dyspnoea, the history is key to distinguishing whether it is of cardiac or respiratory origin. As a general rule, a respiratory history may have associated symptoms such as cough, wheeze, haemoptysis, a smoking history or a relevant occupational history. Likewise, cardiac pathology may have associated symptoms such as palpitations and angina as in this scenario. Examination is also likely to yield collateral findings which will point one towards the cardiac or respiratory system. For example, peripheral oedema is more likely to be associated with cardiac pathology and a barrel shaped chest is more likely to be associated with respiratory pathology. In this case, peripheral oedema may be related to heart failure, varicose veins or be a side effect of the calcium channel blocker. Hypothyroidism is also a cause of peripheral oedema.

It is important to remember that patients may have dual pathology. Smoking causes both cardiovascular and respiratory disease.

Table 1. New York Heart Association Grading of Dyspnoea

Class I No limitations. Ordinary physical activity does not cause undue fatigue, dyspnoea or palpitations.
Class II Slight limitation of physical activity. Ordinary physical activity results in fatigue, palpitations, dyspnoea or angina pectoris.
Class III Marked limitation of physical activity. Less than ordinary physical activity leads to symptoms.
Class IV Unable to carry out any physical activity without discomfort. Symptoms of chronic heart failure present at rest.

Note; the grading allows for symptoms other than that of dyspnoea, thus broadening functional applicability.
Other classifications are described but the above is the commonest in everyday use.

Dyspnoea is a subjective symptom. However, we have means by which we can describe it objectively. Dyspnoea is graded in relation to functional capacity. This allows assessment of its severity and of the disease process and also allows monitoring of its progress. The commonest grading system is that as described by the New York Heart Association.

Cardiac Murmurs

Murmurs may be faint or difficult to hear. Manoeuvres can be performed to allow us to hear them more easily e.g. mitral stenosis is heard better if the patient is turned on his/her left side and the apex is auscultated in this position. In this patient, the murmur of aortic incompetence is best heard at the lower left sternal border with the patient leaning forward in expiration. The patient is asked to hold his breath in expiration (to limit any respiratory/airway sounds as a confounding factor). These manoeuvres aim to reduce the distance between the pathological sound and the stethoscope thereby enabling better auscultation.

Systolic murmurs are easier to hear than diastolic murmurs. They are generally exacerbated by exercise. The patient can be exercised (within limits) to demonstrate these murmurs more clearly. Diastolic ("filling") murmurs are sometimes best interpreted as the absence of the expected silence during ventricular filling.

In this patient, the left ventricular apex is easily felt and displaced to the left due to pathological hypertrophy and dilatation of the ventricle in aortic stenosis. Left ventricular hypertrophy may give rise to a left ventricular heave and a third heart sound. A third heart sound is akin to listening to the hoof sounds of a galloping horse and occurs when the stiffened, less compliant ventricle is filled in diastole. Left ventricular dilatation displaces the apex towards the axilla. A right ventricular heave is felt at the left sternal border with the base of the palm. These signs are subjective. However, repeated clinical experience will allow pattern recognition which is a fundamental pillar of clinical practice.

The patient's narrowed pulse pressure is more consistent with aortic stenosis than aortic incompetence.

Angina

Angina is a symptom of cardiac ischaemia. However, it is not always described by the patient as chest pain. It is often described as a 'tightness' or 'heaviness' and/or an unusual sensation in the praecordium (anterior chest). It most commonly occurs in the praecordium. However, due to the phenomenon of referred pain, it may be felt in the neck, jaw, upper limb, upper epigastrium or posteriorly. Symptoms most commonly are referred on the left hand side, however, they may be bilateral. Diabetics may not have the classical symptom of angina due to autonomic neuropathy. The characteristic diagnosic features of angina are that of exacerbation by exercise and relief by rest and/or glycerol trinitrate. In this patient with aortic stenosis and aortic regurgitation. angina occurs due to a reduced coronary perfusion pressure during diastole thus reducing myocardial oxygen supply. Myocardial oxygen demand may also be increased secondary to the pathological changes which occur with aortic stenosis e.g. left ventricular hypertrophy and left ventricular dilatation.

Symptoms and signs of heart failure are easily conceptualised as either right or left sided in origin. In practice, there is considerable overlap. Symptoms primarily relate to functional limitation as previously described.

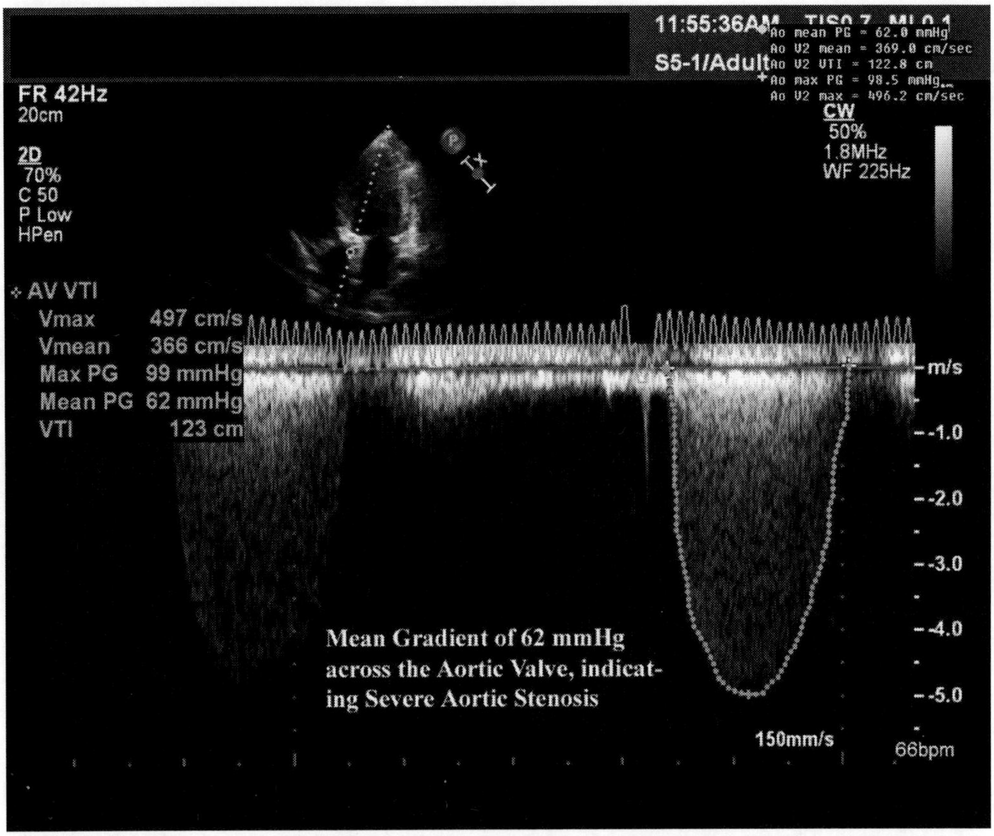

Figure 2. Mean gradient across the Aortic Valve in Severe Aortic Stenosis.
(Photograph courtesy of Mr Saleem Jahangeer, Department of Cardio-Thoracic Surgery, Cork University Hospital, Cork).

The Commonest Cause of Right Heart Failure Is Left Heart Failure

Common Signs of Cardiac Failure

Left

- Tachypnoea
- Basal crepitations
- Cardiomegaly
- Murmurs or added sounds

Right

- Right Ventricular Heave
- Raised JVP
- Hepatomegaly/Ascites
- Peripheral oedema

In this patient, the JVP was raised, but not pathologically so. JVP is assessed with the patient at an angle of 45 degrees. This is the reference point for interpreting a raised JVP. A JVP of greater than 3 cm is regarded as pathological. Observation and interpretation of a raised JVP can be subtle. Carotid pulsation is the obvious misinterpretation. However, carotid pulsation is palpable and is a simpler observable vibration. At the bedside, firm but gentle pressure in the right upper quadrant for a period of time makes the JVP more prominent and therefore easier to identify (hepatojugular reflux or abdominojugular reflux). Contrary to some clinical skills textbooks, interpretation of wave-form within the JVP is generally neither accurate nor informative.

A hepar (hepatomegaly) is a sign of advanced right ventricular heart failure. There needs to be significant tricuspid incompetence to allow chronic congestion of the liver and corresponding hepatomegaly to develop.

Peripheral oedema is a sign of cardiac failure but has a number of causes. In this patient the oedema it is likely to be a combination of cardiac failure and varicose veins. Calcium channel blockers can also cause peripheral oedema. They are also the likely cause of this patient's cool peripheries.

Common Causes of Peripheral Oedema

- Cardiac failure
- Renal failure
- Hepatic failure
- Immobility
- Varicose Veins
- Post Thrombotic limb
- Pregnancy
- Obesity
- Hypoproteinemia
- Drugs
- Hypothyroidism
- Lymphoedema
- Allergy

Observation in a patient with cardiac pathology is very relevant. As in all aspects of clinical examination, observation is highly productive in terms of providing clues relating to aetiology, severity or exacerbating factors. In a patient with cardiac pathology, one may see xanthelasma or corneal deposits of hypercholesterolaemia. Anaemia may be evident (exacerbating or aetiological factor for cardiac pathology). A patient with aortic incompetence may have features of Marfan's syndrome or a patient with longstanding rheumatic mitral stenosis may have reddened cheeks (mitral facies).

Functional observation is extremely helpful if you have the opportunity to perform same. In this patient there was evidence of dyspnoea on mobilisation to the examination couch (NYHA III). The opportunity to walk/exercise with a patient is equally informative (see later).

Lab Spot

Laboratory investigations are helpful in identifying exacerbating factors and possible sequelae of aortic stenosis.

Anaemia is an exacerbating factor. Rarely a haemolytic anaemia develops secondary to red cell membrane fragility. This can occur with intravascular trauma to the red cells as they are ejected in a turbulent fashion through the stenosed aortic valve.

Hyperlipidaemia, hypertriglyceridaemia and lipid protein profile may be identified as contributing factors to coronary artery disease. In this patient, it is important to confirm that she is euthyroid biochemically. Renal profile is necessary as it may reflect cardiac failure or be a cause of peripheral oedema.

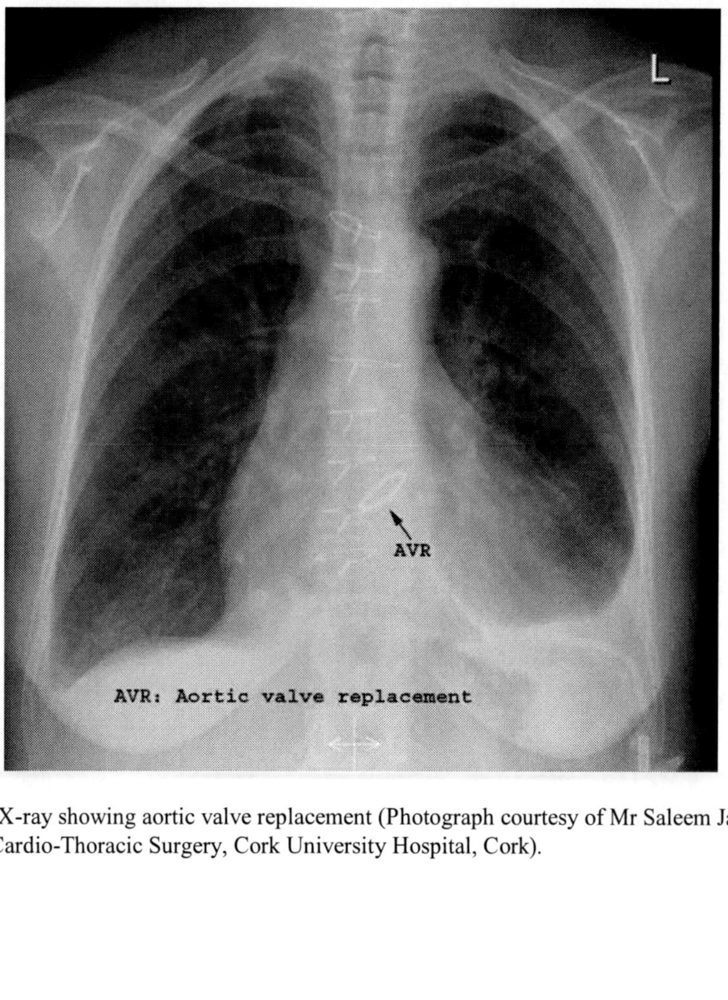

Figure 3. Chest X-ray showing aortic valve replacement (Photograph courtesy of Mr Saleem Jahangeer, Department of Cardio-Thoracic Surgery, Cork University Hospital, Cork).

Pitfalls

1. There is considerable overlap in patients with respiratory and cardiac disease. Dual pathology is very common.
2. Patients who do not experience angina as pain will often not be detected unless leading questions are asked in relation to other subjective symptoms e.g. heaviness, discomfort etc.
3. Women are under diagnosed with cardiac disease as it is sometimes falsely assumed that female gender is fully cardio-protective.
4. Longstanding diabetes may not have classical anginal symptoms.
5. Diastolic murmurs are often missed unless actively looked for.
6. Mild dependent oedema may be evident only in the evening and thus may not be evident during a morning examination. Pitting oedema should primarily be felt (palpated) as distinct from being observed.
7. Thyroid disease is often not thought of as a cause of cardiac disease.

Pearls

1. In a patient with a disease that initially progresses slowly, relatives or those who see the patient intermittently will often provide a more objective assessment of clinical deterioration. Patients can "acclimatise to" their limitations and over time, may regard these as normal.
2. Cardiac symptoms tend to progress in a "snowball fashion". As a snowball rolls down a hill it gets faster and bigger. Likewise with cardiac symptoms -when they develop they tend to progress at an ever increasing speed.
3. Crescendo symptoms (getting more severe and/or frequent) generally flag an impending event e.g. crescendo angina will generally progress to a myocardial infarct. It is vital to identify the pattern within a symptom.
4. The murmur of aortic incompetence is best regarded as the absence of expected silence during diastole at the lower left sternal border.
5. Right heart failure results in hepatomegaly. Hepatomegaly is detected by palpation, percussion and auscultation. In auscultation, the stethoscope is placed over the body of the liver and an oscillating finger is moved from the right lower quadrant ascending to the right upper quadrant. This is a surprisingly accurate means of detecting the liver edge. Remember that it is the liver span that may be abnormal so one needs to percuss the upper edge to define limits. This is particularly relevant in patients with COPD where lung expansion pushes the diaphragm and liver down.
6. Observe from the very start. Observation of the patient as he/she enters the consultation room gives a great deal of information regarding mobility, performance status, discomfort, affect etc.
7. On examining the pulse, the following tip is helpful: press down firmly initially and then ease up slowly until you can feel the pulse at its maximum. It is easier to interpret the rate, rhythm and volume when you do this.

8. Try it. Stethoscope tubing makes and conducts noise. A good way to hear normal and abnormal heart sounds can sometimes be achieved with the patient lying supine and the stethoscope on the chest wall without your hands or the patient being in contact with the tubing. It is noticeably quieter and easier to interpret.
9. As you become more experienced as a clinician, you will not only pause to observe the patient at the beginning of the consultation, but will acutely observe the patient from the beginning to the end of the consultation. The patient's non-verbal responses to your history taking will subtly guide you.

Tips for the OSCE

1. Prepare. Have a mental map or path prepared to execute your examination. In the case of the cardiovascular system you could proceed as follows: 1. General observation › examine the hands › examine the pulse › measure blood pressure › observe and examine face/mouth › examine neck (carotid pulse and JVP) › praecordial examination › abdominal examination hepar/abdominal aorta › peripheral pulses and lower limbs. Once you have a mental path clearly established, it is easier to focus on examination of a particular system.
2. It is good to talk while you are examining. It will make things clearer in your own mind and also allow the examiner to observe that you are covering all relevant areas.
3. Smile and be polite to the patient! Most patients are understandably nervous.
4. Shake the patient's hand. It is good manners and a good way to begin your examination.

Student Check List

- Elicit and grade a history of dyspnoea.
- Elicit a history of angina.
- Know the primary symptoms of Aortic Stenosis.
- Know manoeuvres to amplify a faint murmur.
- Examine a JVP.
- List causes of peripheral oedema.

It Happened to me (It Happens Regularly)

I see both cardiac and thoracic patients at my clinic. Patients in the waiting room are often surprised to see me exiting the consultation room with the patient and heading for the nearest quiet staircase. Both the patient and I walk a number of flights of stairs if appropriate. It provides an accurate, reproducible and objective means to measure cardio-respiratory reserve. A patient may be able to walk one, two or three flights of stairs depending on their cardio-respiratory capacity. Although not very high tech, it can be regarded as a surrogate for the laboratory investigation of maximal oxygen consumption. Once the patient has walked two flights of stairs, I will ask them to recite their name and address and observe whether they can complete same in one sentence. This data is surprisingly robust e.g. patients who can comfortably complete two flights of stairs will generally functionally tolerate a lobectomy as a lung resection. Apart from providing great information, it promotes a rapport between you and the patient and if the clinic is busy it can keep you fit!

> *A few observations and much reasoning lead to error; many observations and a little reasoning to truth.*
>
> Alexis Carrel (Pioneering Surgeon)

In: Learning Clinical Skills
Editors: Bridget Maher and Pat Henn

ISBN: 978-1-62100-409-7

Chapter XIII

Infectious Diseases: A Broad Differential

Mary Horgan, Sarah O'Connell and Sarah Moran

Clinical Case 1

A 21 year old man presented to his GP with a two day history of fevers, fatigue, rash, sore throat and myalgia. He had been well prior to onset of these symptoms. Fevers occur every 6 hours and he feels weak and unwell when his temperature reaches 38 degrees Celsius. He reports having pain on swallowing and swollen, tender neck glands. He denies other associated symptoms including nausea, vomiting or diarrhoea. His appetite has decreased over the past three days. On further questioning, he describes a rash all over his back, trunk and arms. The rash is not itchy and is pink in colour. He checked the rash with the base of a glass yesterday and it disappeared on pressing the glass to his skin.

Past Medical History. Childhood asthma.

Current Medications. Nil. No known drug allergies.

Social History. Accountancy Student. Smoker - 20 cigarettes per day. Alcohol intake: 16 units per week. Shares an apartment with three college friends.

Travel History. He spent the past two months travelling in South East Asia during summer vacation. He reported three episodes of unprotected sexual intercourse with a female in Thailand during this period. He denies intravenous drug during this vacation or otherwise.

Family History. Nil reported.

Review of Systems.

- No joint swelling
- No eye redness or pain
- No dysuria/penile discharge

Clinical Examination

The patient appears well and is in no obvious discomfort. Temperature is 38 degrees C. Blood pressure: 134/76; heart rate 105/minute, regular; oxygen saturations 98% on room air; respiratory rate: 14/min. No scleral icterus present.

Rash -the patient has a macular, pink, blanching rash on his trunk, back and arms. It is diffuse and involves the majority of his skin in these areas. No excoriation or pustules are evident.

Lymph Node Examination -the patient has tender, soft, mobile 2cm. lymphadenopathy in the anterior cervical triangle of neck. Further enlarged lymph nodes are palpable in the right axilla and left submental area.

Respiratory Examination - chest inspection is normal. Chest has normal expansion, there is no tracheal deviation. Percussion is normal. Normal vesicular breath sounds are heard throughout both lungs. No reduction in vocal fremitus and resonance.

Cardiovascular Examination - Heart sounds I and II are clear and audible, with no pericardial rub. JVP is not elevated. No pedal oedema.

Abdominal Examination - the abdomen is soft and non-tender. There are no palpable masses. There is palpable splenomegaly. No palpable hepatomegaly. Multiple mobile non-tender sub-centimetre lymph nodes can be felt in the groin area.

ENT - the patient has white plaque like areas visible on his buccal mucosa and pharynx. There are also some red friable areas where the plaque has been removed. Tonsils are normal in appearance. No visible pustules.

Student Dilemma

1. How do I examine effectively for organomegaly?
2. What are the infectious causes of splenomegaly? (Table 1)
3. Is this infection related to recent travel or not?
4. What tests do I order to reach my diagnosis?
5. What is the diagnostic hallmark of Primary HIV-1 infection?

Discussion

The first important point to note in this history is the patient's age. Given that the majority of young people do not have any co-morbidity, the likelihood is that this illness has occurred de novo. This is an Irish male but he has a history of recent foreign travel. It is always important to take a travel history. The infection that somebody may present with can originate from an endemic area, thus giving clues towards the possible diagnosis.

The patient's rash needs to be a focus of your history-taking. The most important feature to eliminate is whether the rash is blanching or non-blanching. This evaluates petechial rash secondary to meningococcal disease, as this is life threatening and has implications for contact tracing in a university student.

Timing of onset of symptoms is important. Certain infections take a temporal course and can settle with time, for example, in this case, primary HIV-1 infection. If these symptoms had been present for a longer period of time, for example three weeks, and the patient had not been exposed to HIV, this diagnosis would be much less likely.

Lastly, odynophagia is an important part of the history which should not be ignored. In this context it is suggestive of oro-pharyngeal candidiasis secondary to primary HIV-1 infection.

Primary HIV-1 infection is a transient condition, often accompanied by a symptomatic illness of variable severity in 40%-90% of patients. It is invariably accompanied by an initial rapid rise in plasma viraemia and a decrease in the blood $CD4^{+}$ T-cell count and a massive decrease in CD4+ T Cells in the gut and lymph nodes. The signs and symptoms usually appear two-four weeks after virus exposure. The duration of the illness generally lasts between a few days and two weeks. This patient should also undergo full screening for other sexually transitted infections.

Greater than 50% of patients experience myalgia, fatigue, fever, rash and headache. Other symptoms, including pharyngitis, weight loss and arthralgia are experienced to a lesser extent.

Table 1. Infectious Causes of Splenomegaly

- Malaria
- Infective Endocarditis
- Infectious Mononucleosis
- Acute HIV infection
- Chronic HIV Infection
- Chronic Viral Hepatitis B and C complicated by cirrhosis
- Acute Viral Hepatitis
- Epstein Barr Virus
- Cytomegalovirus
- Histoplasmosis
- Schistosomiasis

Table 2. Differential Diagnosis for Primary HIV-1 infection

- Infectious Mononucleosis
- Primary CMV infection
- Enterovirus Meningitis
- Typhoid fever
- Rickettsial infection
- Secondary syphilis

Lab-Spot –Focus on HIV Testing

Anti HIV-1 antibody assays are often negative in the acute phase of illness. Early diagnosis relies on an accurate history of exposure, a positive p24 antigen ELISA (Enzyme-Linked Immunosorbent Assay) or detection of plasma viral RNA by molecular methods. However, the anti HIV-1 antibody assay is a readily available test so should always be performed in the first instance and repeated a few weeks later where there is a clinical suspicion.

Pitfalls

1. Never forget to take a thorough travel and social history.
2. Sexual history is also important and may need to be undertaken in a quiet interview room in a busy Accident and Emergency Department.
3. HIV test is a commonly used and readily available test. Do not be afraid to use it.
4. HIV antibody levels may be negative in primary HIV-1 infection. A negative HIV antibody test does not outrule acute HIV-1 infection.

Pearls

1. A good travel history often points you in the right direction for investigations and diagnosis.
2. Always think of acute HIV infection in any patient that presents with new onset non-specific symptoms including pharyngitis, weight loss, fatigue and headache.
3. Do not assume that certain social classes/ethnicities/heterosexuals are more or less likely to be infected with HIV.

Tips for the OSCE

- When examining for splenomegaly, always ask the patient to lie on his/her right side with their knees drawn up to their chest. This allows for the spleen to hang down from behind the rib cage, allowing palpation of the spleen.
- Perform the full and methodical lymphadenopathy examination.
- Always take a travel, social and sexual history.
- Always check if a rash is blanching or non-blanching before you proceed with other parts of the examination.

Student Check List

- Causes of splenomegaly and how to examine for organomegaly.
- Causes of acute presentation of fever and lymphadenopathy.
- Causes of cervical lymphadenopathy and how to examine for lymphadenopathy.
- Causes of oropharyngeal candidiasis.
- Differential diagnosis of acute HIV-1 infection.
- Know appropriate test for HIV-1 diagnosis in the acute stage of disease.

Clinical Case 2

History

A 20 year old male student is found in his apartment by friends. He is drowsy and acutely unwell. He is brought into hospital by ambulance. He complains of pain on neck flexion, light intolerance and a severe generalized headache. He received empiric antimicrobials from the General Practitioner who reviewed him.

He has no past medical history of note, takes no regular medications, and has no known drug allergies. He is a second year college student and lives with friends. He is a non-smoker and drinks 20 units of alcohol per week.

Examination: Blood pressure is 80/40, heart rate 110bpm, respiratory rate 22/min, Temp 39C, Glasgow Coma Scale (GCS) 13/15 (E3 M4 V6). His peripheries are cold and poorly perfused. A diffuse, non-blanching petechial rash with palpable purpura is noted. There is no evidence of papilloedema. Respiratory, cardiac and abdominal examinations are unremarkable.

Investigations: Computed tomography of brain was performed prior to lumbar puncture and revealed no abnormality. Lumbar puncture was performed and revealed a mildly elevated opening pressure (325mmHg). Cerebrospinal fluid was cloudy and analysis showed an elevated white cell count of 2500/mm with 90% polymorphs, 10% lymphocytes, 0/mm red blood cells, an elevated protein (1370 mg/dl). The CSF: plasma glucose ratio was reduced. Gram stain revealed gram negative diplococci.

Serum investigations revealed an elevated white cell count with left shift, normal renal and liver indices, and elevated C Reactive Protein and Erythrocyte Sedimentation Rate. Blood cultures were taken. Serum samples were sent for PCR. Throat swab was taken.

Diagnosis: Invasive meningococcal disease/meningitis caused by Neisseria meningitides.

Discussion

Diagnosis

Acute bacterial meningitis is classically associated with fever, photophobia, neck stiffness, nausea and vomiting, agitation, headache and altered mental status. Other signs include tachycardia, skin rash and skin discolouration (Figures1, 2).

The differential diagnosis includes viral meningitis, malaria, meningo-encephalitis, septicaemia, subarachnoid haemorrhage, dengue and tetanus.

Management

Meningitis is a medical, neurological and potential neurosurgical emergency. Management is focused on initial general management based on assessment of Airway, Breathing, Circulation and Disability. Specific management includes immediate antimicrobial administration and, in certain cases, steroids.

Airway management involves assessment of level of consciousness (using the Glasgow Coma Scale) to ensure patients have an adequate level of consciousness in order to protect their airway. The Glasgow Coma Scale is scored from a minimum of 3 to a maximum of 15. A score of less than 8 requires anaesthetic management including intubation.

Assessment of breathing includes measurement of respiratory rate, pulse oximetry and the use of high flow oxygen via facemask.

Circulation management includes measurement of heart rate, capillary refill time, the insertion of a wide bore intravenous cannula, fluid resuscitation and measurement of urinary output. In severe cases, inotropic support may be required.

Disability assessment includes full neurological examination (level of consciousness, fundoscopy (papilloedema), power, tone, and cranial nerve examination).

Antibiotics must be administered as soon as possible and should not be delayed by any investigations. Initial therapy should be empirical until the aetiology is established and should include third generation cephalosporin, dexamethasone and vancomycin. Acyclovir should be considered according to the results of the CSF analysis. For uncomplicated meningococcal meningitis, a 7-day course of intravenous ceftriaxone 2g every 12 hours is adequate. If *Listeria monocytogenes* is suspected, amoxicillin 2g intravenously every 4 hours is used. In the case of penicillin allergy, (anaphylaxis only), chloramphenicol and vancomycin should be used.

The use of dexamethasone in the management of bacterial meningitis is controversial; however its adjunctive use may be beneficial.

Prevention of spread requires chemoprophylaxis and immunoprophylaxis. Chemoprophylaxis should be offered to adults in close contact with patients in an endemic situation with a single dose of Ciprofloxacin. Immunoprophylaxis in the form of vaccination can be used for close contacts of patients with meningococcal disease caused by A, C, Y, or W135. The Public Health Department should be notified.

Antibiotics must be administered as soon as possible and should not be delayed by any investigations. The correct antimicrobials depend on local sensitivities. In our institution, first line empiric treatment is intravenous ceftriaxone 2g every 12 hours. If *Listeria Monocytogenes* is suspected, amoxicillin 2g intravenously every 4 hours is used. In the case of penicillin allergy, (anaphylaxis only), chloramphenicol and vancomycin should be used. Treatment should be continued for 7 days in cases of *Neisseria Meningitides* and 10-14 days in case of *Listeria Monocytogenes.*

Investigations

Key investigations include lumbar puncture, blood culture, throat swabs, serum samples for meningococcal and pneumococcal PCR, throat swabs for *Neisseria Meningitides,* serum samples for full blood count, coagulation screen, and liver and renal indices. Lumbar puncture and CSF analysis is used to assess opening pressure (40% of patients with bacterial meningitis have an opening pressure >400 mmHg), cell count (elevated white cell count 10-1000/cmm^3 with a predominance of polymorphs), elevated protein level (usually greater than 50mg/dL), and reduced glucose levels (usually less than 40% of serum levels) (Table 3).

Common Organisms

Neisseria meningitides, Streptococcus Pneumoniae, Haemophilus influenza and *Listeria Monocytogenes.*

Complications

These include hydrocephalus, transtentorial herniation, seizures, stroke, focal cranial nerve palsies, disseminated intravascular coagulopathy and death.

Epidemiology

Neisseria meningitides is found world-wide. There are five major serogroups; A, B, C, W135 and Y. Groups B and C tend to be sporadic and are the commonest in Europe and North America. Groups A, Y and W tend to cause epidemics. Incidence is 1.2 million cases worldwide each year. Meningitis is among the ten most common infectious causes of death and is responsible for approximately 135,000 deaths throughout the world each year. Neurologic sequelae are common among survivors.

At risk populations include early childhood and elderly people with a small peak in adolescents and early adults. There is a seasonal variation with increase in early spring and winter.

Up to 10% of people may carry *Neisseria Meningitides*. Peak carriage rates occur in 15-19 year olds (25%). Carriage is typically followed by the development of immunity. *Neisseria Meningitides* Group C was commonest in Ireland before vaccination was introduced in 2000; Group B now causes 80-85% of meningitis in Ireland at present.

Vaccination

A vaccination programme was introduced in Ireland in October 2000. The vaccine in use in Ireland only protects against *Neisseria Meningitides* Group C. It has reduced the rate of

Neisseria Meningitides Group C meningitis in Ireland from 30-40% to 5% of meningococcal disease per annum. The vaccination programme was initially introduced in infants and then extended to people aged up to 22 years of age. It is also used as prophylaxis treatment for household contacts, close contacts and clustered outbreaks.

Summary

Bacterial meningitis is a common, treatable, potentially fatal illness characterized by fever, headache, rash and neck stiffness. The mainstay of treatment is immediate appropriate antimicrobials.

Student Dilemma

1. Should I give antibiotics before the lumbar puncture?
2. Does everyone need a CT scan prior to lumbar puncture?
3. Is meningococcal meningitis a notifiable disease?
4. How do you contract it?
5. What is a close contact and what prophylaxis should they receive?

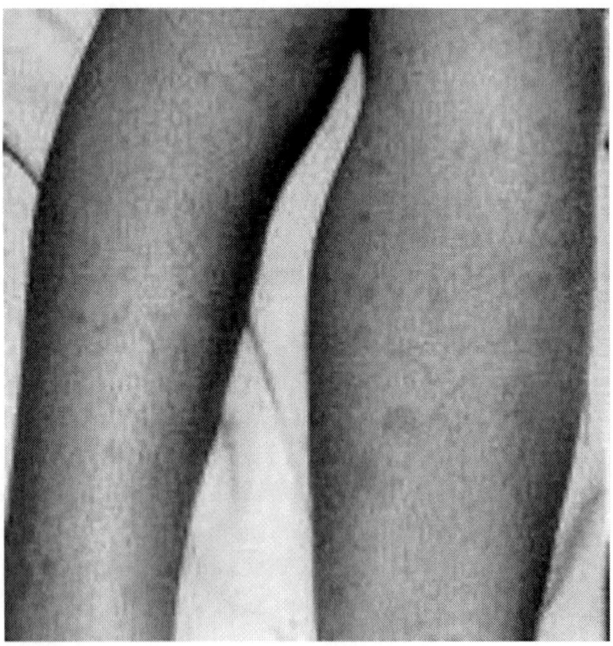

Figure 1. Non-blanching rash.
(Reproduced by kind permission of Meningitis Research Foundation Ireland)

Answers

1. Yes, there should be no delay in administration of antimicrobial therapy. Imaging and lumbar puncture should not delay antibiotics.
2. No, not everyone needs a CT prior to lumbar puncture. CT should be performed if there is clinical suspicion of raised intracranial pressure or if there is diagnostic uncertainty.
3. Yes, meningitis is a notifiable disease in Ireland.
4. Meningitis is contracted by respiratory droplet spread.
5. A close contact is someone who has been sleeping or eating within close contact of the patient e.g. family, day care contacts, girlfriend/boyfriend. Healthcare workers may also be included where they perform invasive procedures on the patient e.g. intubation.

Lab Spot

Table 3. Focus on CSF Analysis

	Normal	**Viral**	**Pyogenic**	**Tuberculosis**
Appearance	Clear and colourless	Clear/ turbid	Turbid/ purulent	Turbid/ purulent
Mononuclear cells	< 5 mm^3	10-100mm^3	<50mm^3	100-300mm^3
Polymorph cells	Nil	Nil	200-300/mm^3	Variable
Protein (mg/dL)	15-40	<100	>100	Normal or raised
Glucose	Normal	>50% plasma	<50% plasma	<50% plasma

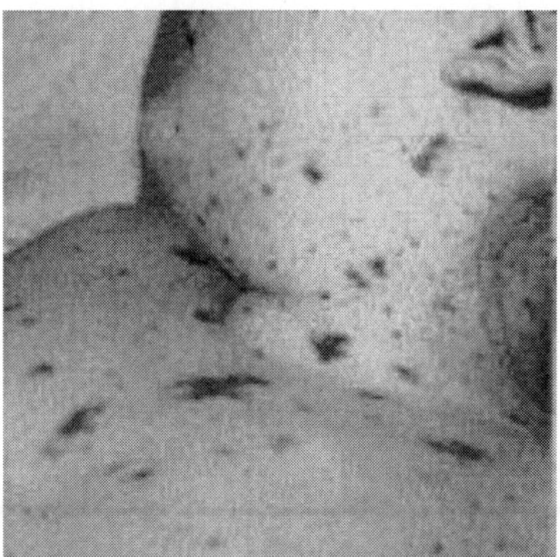

Figure 2. Non-blanching purpuric rash.
(Reproduced by kind permission of Meningitis Research Foundation Ireland)

Pearls

1. If the diagnosis of meningitis is suspected, empiric antibiotics should be given without time delay.
2. Airway, Breathing and Circulation management is the correct approach to the patient with suspected meningitis.
3. Always take a history of close contacts so that prophylaxis can be administered where necessary.

Pitfalls

1. Not all cases of bacterial meningitis are associated with a characteristic rash and meningitis should be suspected even in the absence of a rash.
2. Always take a history for symptoms of raised intracranial pressure and perform a CT scan prior to performing a lumbar puncture. Failure to do this before performing lumbar puncture increases the risk of tentorial herniation in the setting of raised intracranial pressure.
3. If CSF cultures and blood cultures do not reveal any organism, this may signify partially treated bacterial meningitis, and should be treated as such.

'The germ is nothing; the terrain is everything.'

Louis Pasteu

Further Reading

Van de Beek D, de Gans J, Spanjaard L, Weisfeld M, Reitsma JB, Vermeulen M. Clinical features and prognostic factors in adults with bacterial meningitis. N Engl J Med 2004;351:1849-59.

In: Learning Clinical Skills
Editors: Bridget Maher and Pat Henn
ISBN: 978-1-62100-409-7

Chapter XIV

Chronic Kidney Disease Uncovered

Liam Plant

Case History 1

A 37 year old female has CKD Stage 4, with eGFR 22ml/min/1.73m^2. She has well controlled BP at 120/70 (on ACE), with 2.5g/day proteinuria. ECF volume is well controlled by diet and diuretics. She has anaemia, which is corrected by erythropoeitin. She has no evidence of heart failure. In anticipation of needing dialysis, she has a functioning left forearm AV fistula. Having had Type I diabetes, with proliferative retinopathy, for 23 years, her cause of CKD is diabetic nephropathy. The long-term management plan is to target her for a simultaneous kidney-pancreas transplant.

Case History 2

This 76 year old male has CKD Stage 5, with eGFR 9ml/min/1.73m^2. BP is poorly controlled at 176/103, with evidence of an expanded ECF volume (oedema; pulmonary oedema; pleural effusions). He has a muddy-brown complexion, with pale mucous membranes (and is not on erythropoietin). He has a uraemic foetor, frequent myoclonic jerks and is drowsy. He has just been referred to Renal Services.

Discussion

Chronic Kidney Disease (CKD) is common, afflicting up to 10% of adults. It has many causes (diabetic nephropathy, glomerular disease, chronic pyelonephritis, autosomal dominant polycystic kidney disease, amyloidosis, multi-system disease, etc.) It is commonly progressive, and the clinical features and associated complications become more extensive as renal function declines. It is best evaluated generically; then stratified into stages.

CKD exists if a patient has *at least one* of the following features:

- Persistent proteinuria
- Persistent haematuria, not due to UTI, urological tumour, urolithiasis
- Persistent radiological abnormality of the kidney(s)
- Persistent histological abnormality of the kidney(s)

Or, *in the absence of these,* a persistent estimated Glomerular Filtration Rate (eGFR) $<60ml/min/1.73m^2$, when assayed in a clinically stable outpatient/GP surgery environment.

Once it is established that CKD exists, then the cardinal features (which should always inform the initial description of the status of all patients with CKD) include:

- *Hypertension,* which occurs in over 85% of cases. Systolic hypertension is especially prominent, often with other signs of target organ damage such as left ventricular hypertrophy (LVH) – which can be confirmed by ECG or echocardiography. Retinal changes of hypertension may be seen with dilated fundoscopy (a key evaluation) – Keith-Wagener Stage III/IV changes (haemorrhages/exudates or papilloedema) indicate accelerated phase hypertension. Higher blood pressure increases the rate of decline of renal function and increases the probability of other cardiovascular complications.
- In CKD, a target BP of <130/80 should be attained in all patients; patients of African, South Asian or Aboriginal ethnic origins, or with protein excretion >3g/day, should achieve a target BP of <125/75.
- *Proteinuria,* which is a further predictor of progression and of the development of complications (particularly if combined with poorly controlled hypertension). Reagent strip dipstick urinalysis is used to screen for proteinuria (ideally in an early morning sample). If detected on screening, proteinuria can (and should) be quantified, either by 24-hr urinary protein excretion collection or spot urinary protein-creatinine ratio. Urinary *albumin* excretion requires a more specific assay (either reagent strip Albustix®; 24-hr urinary albumin excretion; or spot urinary albumin-creatinine ratio) and is principally used in the detection and monitoring of incipient diabetic nephropathy.
- A 24-hr protein excretion of >300mg/day, or spot protein-creatinine ratio >35mg/mmol, is the conventional threshold used for defining 'proteinuria'. A 24-hr albumin excretion of 30-300mg/day, or spot albumin-creatinine ratio of 3.5-35mg/mmol, defines 'microalbuminuria'.
- *eGFR* is widely estimated from 4 variables – age, gender, race and stable serum [creatinine] – using the modified MDRD equation. Although not as precise as isotope methods, it is more reliable than creatinine clearance estimations based on 24-hr urine collection.

When the level of eGFR has been established, 5 stages of stratification are established:

1. eGFR >90ml/min/1.73m^2
2. eGFR 60-89ml/min/1.73m^2
3. eGFR 30-59ml/min/1.73m^2
4. eGFR 15-29ml/min/1.73m^2
5. eGFR <15ml/min/1.73m^2

Within the above framework, diagnosis and the detection of complications can proceed.

Underlying Causes of CKD

History and examination may offer clues as to why a patient has developed CKD. Long-standing Type I diabetes, especially with other features of microvascular disease such as proliferative retinopathy, and especially if there has been poor metabolic control, may progress through microalbuminuria to proteinuria to progressive CKD. The nephropathy of Type II diabetes may follow a shorter history of diabetes, and macrovascular complications are often present from an early stage. In both of these causes, proteinuria is a prominent feature. Renal biopsy shows characteristic histology, but is rarely required in the context of a suggestive history,

Primary glomerular diseases such as IgA nephropathy, membranous nephropathy, and focal segmental glomerulosclerosis (FSGS) are common causes of CKD. Such patients may pass through a phase of Nephrotic Syndrome (oedema, proteinuria, hypoalbuminaemia) – as may patients with diabetic nephropathy. Haematuria and proteinuria are the cardinal features of glomerular disease. Renal biopsy may be necessary to evaluate the specific type of glomerular disease.

A history of urinary tract infection in early childhood, particularly if there is documented evidence of renal scarring or significant vesico-ureteric reflux on imaging, may underlie later CKD. Complicated renal stone disease may also lead to chronic pyelonephritis. In older adults, especially men with symptoms of prostatism, obstructive uropathy may lead to progressive CKD. Clinical examination for an enlarged bladder is important, as is digital rectal examination, PSA assessment and renal tract ultrasonography.

Family history may offer further clues. A history of End Stage Kidney Disease (ESKD) with an autosomal dominant inheritance pattern suggests Autosomal Dominant Polycystic Kidney Disease (ADPKD). Abdominal examination, which should involve the technique of *balloting,* may reveal enlarged kidneys (and liver). Some families will also have a history of sub-arachnoid haemorrhage/intra-cerebral aneurysms. Occasional patients will have the bruit of mitral valve prolapse. A family history of kidney disease with an X-linked inheritance pattern, and a history of deafness, suggests Alport Syndrome. Renal ultrasonography helps confirm the diagnosis of ADPKD.

Some patients may have the clinical features and laboratory features of particular multi-system diseases such as SLE, rheumatoid arthritis, Wegener's Granulomatosis, and multiple myeloma, in which renal involvement is common. Autoimmune serologies, serum complement levels, serum and urine electrophoresis and renal biopsy may be necessary to confirm these diagnoses.

Increasingly, CKD may be a manifestation of atheromatous renal vascular disease, occurring in tandem with clinical evidence of ischaemic heart disease, peripheral vascular disease, carotid artery disease or cerebrovascular disease. This relationship is bi-directional: patients with CKD have dramatically increased frequencies of symptomatic macrovascular disease at other sites.

General Clinical Features

As a general rule of thumb, the more advanced the stage of CKD, the more prominent the clinical complications. Many patients with CKD Stage 3 (particularly if they are on appropriate medications) will be essentially asymptomatic, with well controlled hypertension and only minor proteinuria.

- Extra-Cellular Fluid (ECF) Overload

  As renal function deteriorates, and especially if significant reduction in dietary salt intake has not occurred, an expansion of ECF volume occurs in the majority of patients. This is initially manifest as hypertension (and can increase the possibility that hypertension may enter an accelerated phase). Subsequently, expanded ECF volume is detected by an increase in weight, peripheral oedema, elevated JVP, pleural effusions, pulmonary oedema, ascites (and the characteristic symptoms and signs of these conditions).
- Physical appearance

  The 'traditional' appearance of a patient with CKD is less widely seen in an era of integrated chronic disease management, erythropoietin, dietary manipulation, etc. In patients with long-standing CKD Stage 4-5 (and especially those on dialysis) one may appreciate the typical 'muddy-brown' skin colouration which is attributed to the accumulation of urochromes. In patients not treated with erythropoietin, pallor may be prominent. In those in whom calcium and phosphate homeostasis has not been well controlled, pruritis with excoriations, skin lichenification and nodular prurigo may be encountered. In patients presenting late, with poorly controlled advanced CKD, acidosis may manifest as Kussmaul respiration; there may be an ammoniacal 'uraemic foetor' on the breath; myoclonic jerks and akathesia may be evident. However, such signs will be infrequent in the majority of patients with good chronic disease care pathways.
- Cardiac disease

  The overlap between cardiac disease and renal disease is now much better evaluated, and a variety of 'Cardio-Renal Syndromes' have been defined. Practically all patients with CKD will have LVH, and many of these will have evidence of diastolic heart failure. Others will have progressed through cardiac enlargement and dilatation (due to chronic systolic hypertension, uraemia and ischaemic heart disease) to a state of chronic systolic heart failure. The commonest mode of cardiac death in patients with CKD is not ischaemia/myocardial infarction, but heart failure. Careful clinical evaluation for evidence of heart failure is a very important element of the history and examination in these patients. This is often difficult in the presence of an expanded ECF predominantly due to low GFR, and concomitant renal anaemia (the signs and symptoms will be very similar). A minority of patients, typically those presenting late to Renal Services, develop uraemic pericarditis and may have a typical pericardial 'rub' on auscultation, and possible pericardial effusion with tamponade.

- Anaemia, iron deficiency, secondary hyperparathyroidism

  These are practically universal features in patients with CKD Stage 4-5, and are best tracked with laboratory values. In contemporary healthcare, they will often be well managed, with few symptoms. However, many patients presenting late will initially manifest the cardinal symptoms of anaemia. Some may also present with proximal myopathy (due to the combination of uraemia, secondary hyperparathyroidism, vitamin D deficiency).

Clinical Features in ESKD

End-Stage Kidney Disease exists where a patient remains alive because of the use of long-term renal replacement therapy (dialysis or renal transplant). This is not a common group of patients (typically with a prevalence of 800-1000 p.m.p. in developed societies). These patients are encountered more frequently in Teaching Hospital environments. Patients treated with different forms of renal replacement therapies may have characteristic clinical features, as well as the general features of kidney disease.

- Haemodialysis patients

  Patients may have evidence of current or previous Arterio-Venous fistulae (either native or utilising subcutaneous PTFE loops). These may be on either forearm ('radio-cephalic') or upper arm ('brachio-cephalic'/'brachio-basilic'). Functioning AV fistulae can be identified by their palpable thrills and audible bruits on auscultation. Some haemodialysis patients have 'tunnelled lines' for dialysis vascular access, typically placed in the internal jugular vein and tunnelled out below the clavicle. If infected, the exit site may be erythematous, swollen or purulent.

- Peritoneal dialysis patients

  These patients have indwelling peritoneal catheters, tunnelled out subcutaneously to the lower abdomen. Exit sites can be chronically or acutely infected. In the presence of peritonitis, purulent dialysate with a 'cloudy' appearance will be drained.

- Renal Transplant recipients

  These patients may have skin features of steroid use, or perhaps hirsutism and gum hypertrophy due to ciclosporin use (again, these features are less common in contemporary practice). Signs/scars of previous access for dialysis may be found. Skin lesions are common in these patients (as a consequence of long-standing immunosuppression). These will range from simple viral warts, through actinic keratoses, basal cell carcinomata and squamous cell carcinomata. Renal transplants are typically placed in the right or left iliac fossae and can be palpated. Auscultation will reveal renal artery bruits in a proportion. Anaesthesia/dysaesthesia of the ipsilateral medial or lateral cutaneous nerves of the thigh may be detected in the early stages after a transplant procedure.

Lab-Spot

- Proteinuria - 24-hr urinary protein excretion of >300mg/day, or spot urinary protein-creatinine ratio >35mg/mmol.
- Microalbuminuria - 24-hr urinary albumin excretion of 30-300mg/day, or spot urinary albumin-creatinine ratio of 3.5-35mg/mmol.

Pearls

- In very thin patients, the lower pole of a normal right kidney may be palpable.
- Always observe the macroscopic appearance of a urine sample – is it cloudy, frothy (protein), abnormal colour?
- CKD is often an insidious disease – many patients are asymptomatic. Fatigue is common, but hypertension is even more common.

Tips for the OSCE

In Patients with Renal Disease -

- Don't forget to check for sacral oedema.
- Know how to ballot the kidneys.
- Always perform fundoscopy if BP is quite elevated.
- Check for peripheral neuropathy.
- Always check for abdominal bruits (renal artery stenosis).

'Seeing is an Art that must be Learned'

Leonardo Da Vinci

In: Learning Clinical Skills
Editors: Bridget Maher and Pat Henn

ISBN: 978-1-62100-409-7

Chapter XV

The Older Patient

Denis O'Mahony

Clinical Case 1

An 85 year old female presents with a 5 day history of confusion, new-onset urinary incontinence and faecal soiling. She has a history of hypertension, osteoarthritis, constipation and depression. She was recently commenced on co-codamol for her arthritis pain and also regularly takes verapamil, lactulose and dothiepin for her other chronic conditions. Collateral history from her daughter indicates that the patient's mood and cognitive function were normal prior to the onset of her present confusional state and that she was functionally independent for all activities of daily living.

On examination, the patient is confused and agitated and therefore, unable to give a clear account of her symptoms. Vital signs are as follows: BP 162/94; heart rate 84/min., regular; temperature 37.8^{0}C; respiratory rate 18/min.

Abdominal examination reveals a mass to deep palpation in the left iliac fossa and a second smooth, tender mass in the suprapubic area, arising from the pelvis. The second mass is dull to precussion. Rectal examination reveals faecal impaction and the faecal occult blood test is negative. There are signs of osteoarthritis in both knee joints, the right hip joint, the lumbar spine and both hands. There are no other abnormal clinical signs detectable.

Dipstick urinalysis (catheter sample) reveals 3+ protein, 2+ blood, 3+ nitrite and the sample is malodorous. The catheter drains 1100 ml of urine. Urine microscopy shows copious neutrophils and Gram stain shows a high concentration of Gram negative bacilli.

Lab results are as follows: Haematology - WCC 21.1 10^9/L, Hb 13.2g/dl, Platelets 420 10^9/L; Biochemistry: Na 144 mmol/l, K 5.8 mmol/l, urea 14.3 mmol/l, creatinine 135 mmol/l, C-reactive protein 219 mg/l.

Diagnosis: Urinary tract infection with delirium.

Pathogenesis: Combination of codeine (in co-codamol), verapamil and dothiepin (tricyclic antidepressant with anti-cholinergic effects) leading to severe constipation and faecal impaction of the rectum, leading to bladder outflow obstruction, leading to urinary retention and urinary stasis, predisposing to contamination with intestinal Gram negative organisms, leading to infection. Urinary tract infection is the leading cause of acute confusion (delirium) in older people.

Table 1. Student Dilemma

- How can I make a clinical diagnosis when the patient cannot give a clear history, as in this case of delirium?
- How do I distinguish delirium from dementia?
- Doesn't the patient need an abdominal ultrasound to confirm urinary retention?
- How do I do a digital rectal examination in a confused patient?
- How do I interpret dipstick urinalysis? (see Figure 1)

Discussion

Accurate clinical diagnosis without a clear history from the patient is usually challenging. But, in the 'real world' scenario, some simple tips will help, such as getting a clear collateral history from the patient's spouse, next-of-kin, carer or other person who knows the patient's usual physical and mental status very well and who is best placed to compare the usual status with the present status. Often, a simple phone call is all that is required if the reliable informant is not available. If the informant is on hand, his/her account is invaluable when trying to obtain clinical history details from a confused patient.

Delirium often occurs in older patients with underlying dementia. Whether dementia is concurrently present or not, the typical features of delirium that are not present in dementia are listed in Table 2. The hallmark of delirium is cognitive impairment, which can be quickly and easily measured using the 10-question Abbreviated Mental Test Scale (AMTS – Table 3). Sometimes, however, older patients with delirium may perform well on the AMTS, scoring ≥ 8/10. Therefore, if in doubt, the Mini-Mental State Examination (MMSE – Table 4) is more discriminatory, a score of ≤ 23/30 being considered definitely abnormal.

Delirium is characterized by difficulty with clear communication with the patient. Other causes of impaired communication are listed in Table 5 and are easily called to mind by remembering the letter 'D'.

Table 2. The Clinical Characteristics of Delirium

- Impaired attention
- Impaired cognition in more than one domain
- Altered level of alertness, from drowsy (hypoactive delirium) to agitated (hyperactive delirium)
- Fluctuating course within a 24 hour period
- Onset over hours to days

Table 3. Abbreviated Mental Test Scale (AMTS)

1. What is your age?
2. What is the time (to the nearest hour)?
3. What is the year?
4. What place is this?
5. Simple address for recall at the end of the test (e.g. 42, North Street)
6. Identify two persons correctly (e.g. nurse, other doctor)
7. What is your date of birth?
8. In what year did the Second World War began?
9. Who is the current President of Ireland?
10. Count backwards from 20 to 1.

Guide: 9/10 or 10/10 normal; 8/10 borderline; ≤ 7/10 abnormal.

Urinary retention is usually an easy clinical diagnosis: a smooth, ovoid mass arising from the pelvis, dull to percussion, usually tender to palpation if urinary retention is acute. Urinary incontinence does not exclude the diagnosis, as overflow dribbling incontinence is not uncommon with urinary retention. The diagnosis does not depend on the patient having a bladder ultrasound, simply passing a urinary catheter will both confirm the diagnosis (large volume, i.e. usually > 500 ml drainage of urine within 5 minutes) and relieve the pain and distress of acute urinary retention.

Table 4. Mini-Mental State Examination (MMSE)

A. What is the day (1), time (1), Month (1), year (1), Season (1); subscore ..../5
B. Name of this place (1), district (1), town (1), street/road nearest to home (1), county (1); subscore: ..../5.
C. Registration of 3 simple nouns: Ball:...(1); Flag: ...(1); Tree: ...(1); number of attempts:......... ; subscore: ..../3
D. Mental arithmetic: Subtract serial 7's from 100: 93 (1); 86 (1); 79 (1); 72 (1); 65 (1); subscore: ..../5
E. Recall of 3 words Ball:...(1); Flag: ...(1); Tree: ...(1); subscore: ..../3
F. Recognition of 2 objects: Wristwatch: ....(1); Pen: .....(1); subscore: ..../2 Sentence repetition: 'No ifs, ands or buts'(1): ....
G. 3 stage command: 'Take this piece of paper in your right hand'(1): ....; 'Fold it in half'(1): .....; 'Place it on the table in front of you'(1): .....; subscore: ..../3
H. Look at this command and do what it says: CLOSE YOUR EYES (1): ....
I. Write a short sentence with a noun and a verb in it (1): ....
J. Copy this drawing (two intersecting pentagons; 1): ....

Guide: Maximum score 30/30; 23/30 or less indicates definite cognitive impairment. Allow for possible visual or hearing impairment and mark accordingly.

Table 5. Causes of impaired communication in older people

- Dysphasia: disorder of language formulation or comprehension.
- Dysarthria: disorder of articulation.
- Dysphonia: disorder of vocal cord volume.
- Delirium: disorder of cognition, attention (acute)
- Dementia: disorder of cognition with normal sensorium (chronic)
- Deafness

Digital rectal examination (DRE), whilst often difficult to perform in a confused patient, is nevertheless the most important clinical test for faecal impaction and assessment of prostate gland size and contour in males. If a patient has suspected urinary retention and is in distress, it is always better to pass a urinary catheter to relieve the urinary retention first and wait until the patient is more comfortable before progressing to DRE. DRE in the confused, elderly patient is invariably best approached with the assistance of an experienced nurse or doctor to reassure and explain to the patient what is being done and why. If the patient is severely agitated, it is best to defer the DRE until he/she is not agitated, and is calmer and more amenable to the DRE.

Dipstick urinalysis is a simple but important skill for all medical and nursing staff (Figure 1). The dipstick essentially represents a series of colour changes that occur in response to the presence of erythrocytes, leucocytes, proteinuria > 1g/l, conjugated bilirubin, urobilinogen, nitrite and changes in specific gravity. Urinary tract infection (UTI) is highly likely when erythrocytes, leucocytes, proteinuria and nitrites are detected simultaneously. Also, the characteristic 'fishy' odour and turbid appearance of infected urine help point towards a diagnosis of UTI.

Lab-spot

Focus on Mid-stream Specimen of Urine (MSU) Reports in Adults

Microbiology laboratories report urine microscopy and culture results as follows:

i) Number of red cells per ml
ii) Number of leucocytes per ml
iii) Presence of visible crystals or tubular casts
iv) Number of organisms per ml
v) Antibiotic sensitivities after 24 hour exposure to a selection of typical antibiotics commonly used to treat urinary tract infection (UTI)

For example, an MSU report may read as follows:

Erythrocytes: 40 per ml

Leucocytes: > 500 per ml
Organisms: 10^5 coliforms per ml
Sensitivities: Trimethoprim R Ampicillin R

Nitrofurantoin S	Gentamicin S	S = sensitive
Cephradine S	Ciprofloxacin S	R = resistant

Interpretation: This is a proven coliform (Gram negative) UTI. Appropriate treatment would be nitrofurantoin, gentamicin, cephradine or ciprofloxacin (the coliform organism is sensitive to these antibiotics); trimethoprim and ampicillin-based antibiotics e.g. amoxicillin should be avoided, since the coliform organism is resistant to these antibiotics.

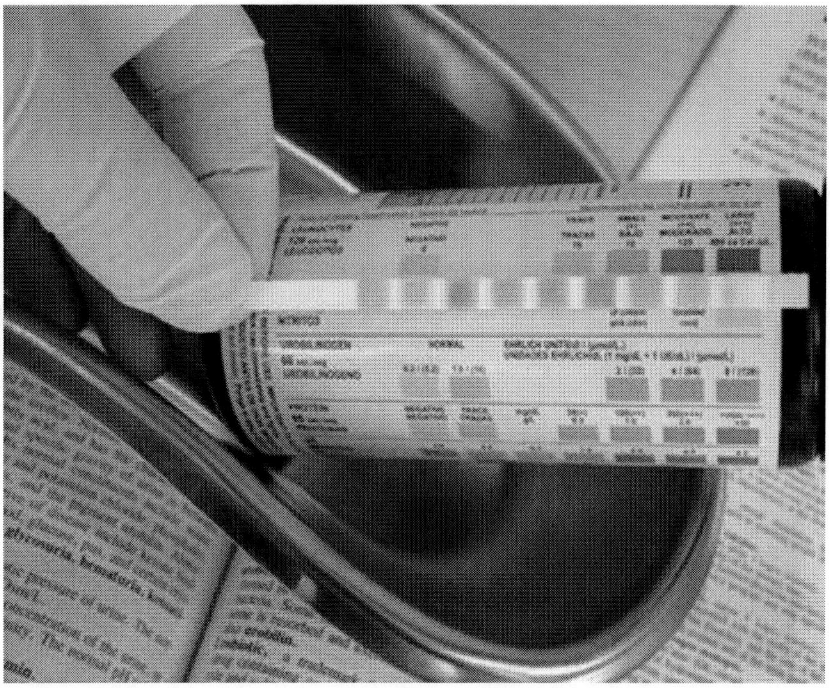

Figure 1. Dipstick urinalysis is a simple, but essential clinical skill. It provides instant diagnostic information.

Pitfalls in Older Patient Assessment

Pitfall 1: Describing the Patient as a 'Poor Historian'

Never forget: *you* are the historian, not the patient. If the older patient is not giving you a clear, precise account of his/her symptoms, there is always an important reason i.e. one of the 6D's referred to in Table 5. If the patient cannot give a clear, accurate description of symptoms and previous medical history because of, say, dementia, you must switch to *collateral* history-taking, i.e. obtaining details from family members, the patient's GP, home help, public health nurse etc. Calling the patient a 'poor historian' is unfair scape-goating of the patient.

Pitfall 2: Opting for a 'Limited Examination'

Never yield to the temptation of performing a 'limited examination' in an older patient just because a full examination is challenging; you will very likely miss important physical signs. Get the necessary help of a clinical colleague or a relative and make sure that both you and the patient are comfortable before proceeding. In particular, do not avoid performing a digital rectal examination where it is clearly indicated (e.g. urinary retention, rectal bleeding). You will likely miss diagnostic signs, as in the case of older women with acute urinary retention, who usually have faecal impaction causing bladder outflow obstruction.

Pitfall 3: Thinking that it Is 'just Old Age'

Acute illness in old age often presents non-specifically, typically with falls, confusion, incontinence, immobility and 'gone-off' syndrome (i.e. subacute, non-specific deterioration). Each of these classical geriatric syndromes is typically multifactorial; identifying the risk factors for the presenting problem is the key to deciphering it. Careful assessment will identify the relevant risk factors which are often treatable/modifiable, facilitating recovery and rehabilitation. Falls, confusion, incontinence, immobility and 'gone-off' syndrome are not normal in old age and accepting them as 'just old age' is to completely miss the point.

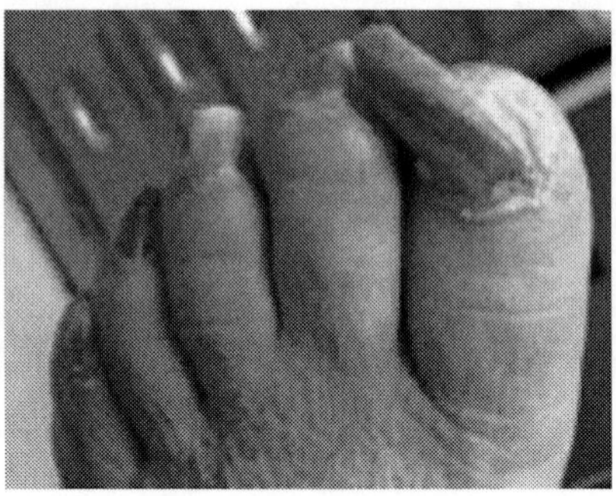

Figure 2. Foot and nail pathology is common in older people. It often signifies self-neglect due to other problems that preclude nail trimming (e.g. severe hip arthritis) or availing of chiropody (e.g. dementia, financial poverty).

Pitfall 4: If you Have to Shout, you're Doing Something Wrong

Deafness is common in late life and is often undiagnosed prior to a patient presenting for assessment. Many older people accept loss of auditory acuity as 'just old age' or may neglect to use their hearing aids properly when treated for true neural sensory deafness. Cerumen impaction of the external auditory canals is very common, so much so that one should assume that this is the cause of deafness until proven otherwise by otoscopy. Cerumen impaction is easy to detect and treat. Otoscopy is one of the quickest and best tolerated diagnostic tests in clinical practice, yet is commonly overlooked/neglected. In cases of established neural sensory deafness, often the communication barrier between patient and doctor is overcome by simply speaking slowly and clearly close to the patient's 'better' ear.

Pitfall 5: If you Miss the Feet, you May Miss the Point

Serious foot pathology is highly prevalent in older people, yet is often overlooked or not detected. Many older people leave their socks on in bed when they feel unwell. Sometimes, personal hygiene is poor and may deter more sensitive doctors from examining the feet. Proper examination of the feet will often identify arthritis, ulceration, peripheral vascular disease, skin pathology and nail disorders (Figure 2).

Also, the state of an elderly patient's feet and toenails informs the doctor with quiet candour whether the patient is suffering from neglect.

Pitfall 6: Failure to Detect Cognitive Impairment Can Be a very Serious Mistake

Cognitive impairment, both of the acute type (delirium) and of the chronic, progressive type (dementia) is highly prevalent in late life. Like recording pulse and blood pressure, documenting a patient's cognition is a fundamental part of elderly patient assessment. Failure to detect cognitive impairment can be catastrophic, e.g. prescribing a medicine with a narrow therapeutic window (e.g. warfarin, insulin) to an older person with undetected dementia living alone or without competent supervision. Early dementia can be very subtle, i.e. present with AMTS and MMSE scores in the 'normal' range i.e. $\geq 8/10$ for the AMTS and $\geq 24/30$ for the MMSE. However, a collateral history of noticeable, progressive loss of short-term memory is a reliable clinical indicator. Also, 'concrete thinking' is a helpful sign; this is demonstrated by inability to give the correct meaning to a series of common proverbs or sayings. However, cognitive screening tests like the AMTS and the MMSE are not *diagnostic* tests for delirium or dementia, merely cognitive assessment tools.

Pearls in Older Patient Assessment

Pearl 1: "We See only what we Look for, we Look for only what we Know"

This was a famous aphorism of Sir William Osler (Figure 3), the father of modern clinical medicine. A broad and mature knowledge base is the foundation for being a competent diagnostician in any field of clinical practice. Nowhere is this more true than in the specialty of Clinical Gerontology. A sound knowledge of the clinical science underpinning Clinical Gerontology and its associated therapeutics is the key to effective clinical practice in older people; without a firm grasp of the clinical science and therapeutics of illness in late life, there will be endless frustration for doctor and patient.

Pearl 2: Slow down to the Older Patient's Pace

Cognitive and sensory deficits in many older people mean that the conversation that forms the basis of the clinical history has to be conducted at a slower pace to be effective. This may mean using deliberately slower speech when asking questions, using shorter sentences and a gentle increase in the volume of your voice. Application of these simple precepts can often be the difference between success and failure when taking a history from an older patient.

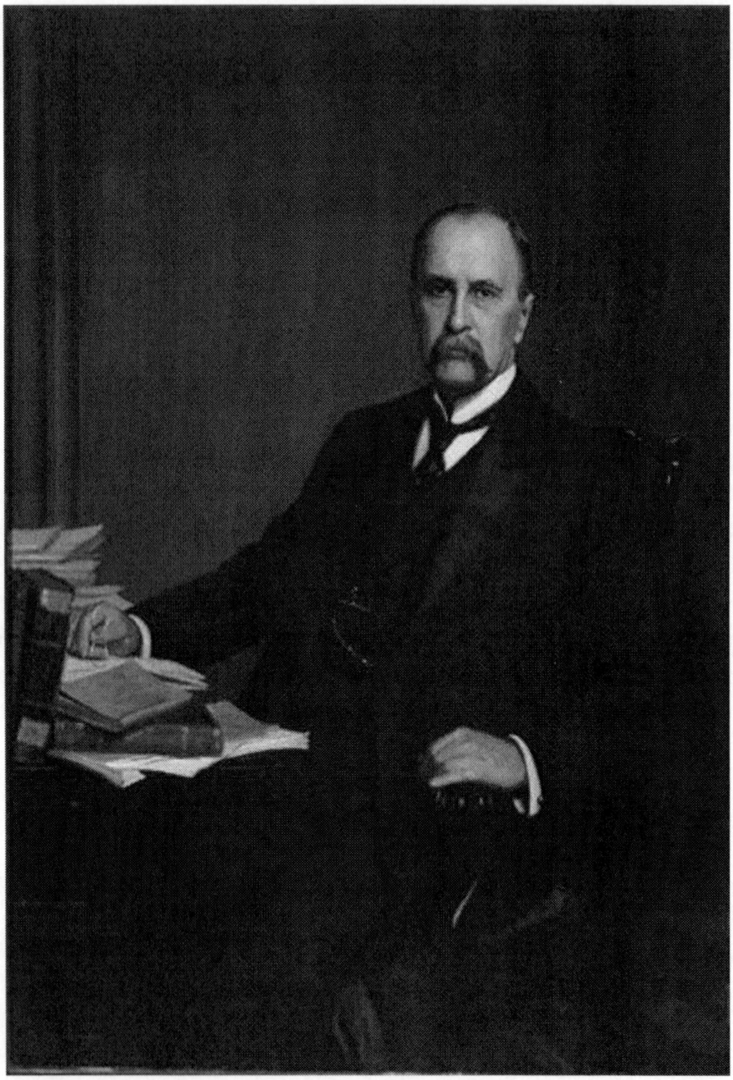

Figure 3. Sir William Osler (1849-1919) was the father of modern clinical medicine. A Canadian, he practiced and taught mostly in Oxford, UK. He constantly emphasised the importance of clinical diagnosis that is based on keen observation and establishing the facts from rigorous history-taking and thorough, skillful clinical examination. His precepts, like those of Hippocrates, are timeless and apply to every generation of medical students and practicing doctors.

Pearl 3: Iatrogenic Illness Is Common in Older People

Older people are the biggest consumers of prescription drugs globally. Iatrogenic illness is highly prevalent in older people, particularly those taking eight or more daily drugs. Multiple comorbidity is the basis of frailty in older people. The multiple medical conditions that form the basis of multiple comorbidity commonly lead to multiple medications, often prescribed by different organ specialists, without due consideration to potential adverse drug-drug interactions and drug-disease interactions. Although adverse drug reactions in older people are usually of the non-idiosyncratic, predictable kind, often the presentation of iatrogenic illness is non-specific, e.g. falls, confusion, incontinence, anorexia. For most illness presentations in older people taking multiple medications, always consider the possibility of iatrogenesis as the whole or part of the diagnosis.

Pearl 4: Multiple Comorbidity Is more the Rule than the Exception, Particularly in those Aged over 80

As we age, chronic ailments accumulate. These chronic disorders predispose to impaired physiological homeostasis and vice versa. Most people aged over 80 have two or more chronic medical problems. Through the ninth decade and beyond, chronic disorders usually accumulate. In general, these chronic disorders are self-evident and easy to detect. Although the disorders (e.g. osteoarthritis, prostatism, hypertension, diabetes, dementia, COPD etc) may appear mundane, understanding their complex interaction and the manifold associated clinical phenomena arising from these complex interactions, is the key to understanding the presentation and progression of illness in late life.

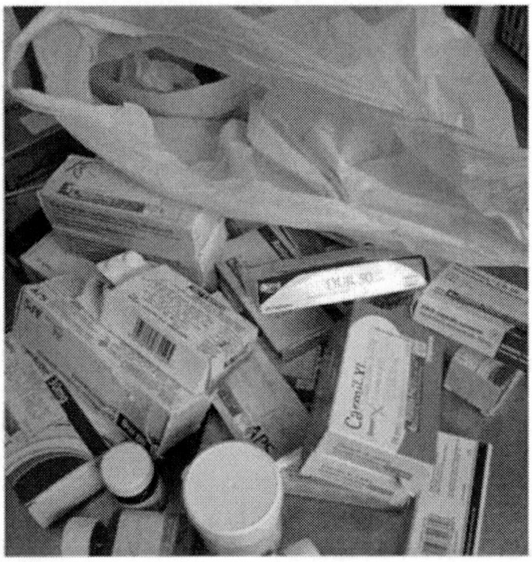

Figure 4: Major polypharmacy is a common finding in older, frailer patients. It often leads to confusion for both patient and doctor. It is also the single greatest risk factor for iatrogenic illness and as such, should be viewed as a health hazard.

Pearl 5: A Detailed, Accurate Drug History Is Crucial

Major polypharmacy i.e. the consumption of 10 or more daily medicines is not uncommon in older people (Figure 4); polypharmacy, in turn, reflects multiple comorbid illnesses (which often signifies overall frailty). Polypharmacy is the single greatest risk factor for adverse drug reactions, a major cause of hospitalization in older people. A detailed, accurate drug history is particularly important in older patients, since they are the biggest consumers of prescription and 'over-the-counter' (OTC) drugs. Ask the patient for all details relating to their medications; if necessary, enquire from the patient's carer/relative/ GP/pharmacist to confirm details. Always ask about herbal and homeopathic medicines; sometimes, these can cause major adverse interactions with the patient's prescription drugs and chronic medical conditions. When taking details of drug allergy (usually manifesting as acute rash, oedema, wheeze or hypotension), also be sure to enquire about drug intolerance, as distinct from allergy (e.g. dyspepsia or gastrointestinal bleeding from consumption of non-steroidal anti-inflammatory drugs). Finally, ask the patient to show you their drugs; this can be very revealing, as what is actually consumed may be at variance with the drug list in the patient's medical or pharmacy records.

Pearl 6: The Prioritized Clinical Problem List Helps Focus the Mind

In older patients, particularly frailer ones, summarizing their cases with prioritized problem lists is usually helpful. Typically, frailer older people have a multiplicity of chronic disorders, with one or more of these conditions causing the presenting symptoms. However, one cannot ignore the other chronic disorders, since they usually have a bearing on the clinical progress and management of the patient. Using a prioritized problem list allows the doctor, at a glance, to review the patient's medical status and to make appropriate choices in management of that patient quickly. Furthermore, if a doctor who is not familiar with an older patient with complex co-morbidity needs to review the patient (e.g. whilst working an on-call shift), having the patient's up-to-date prioritized problem list is invaluable.

Pearl 7: The Social History Must be Detailed and Diverse

All too often, older patients' social history contains details of their marital status, tobacco and alcohol consumption and nothing more. One must include details of previous occupation(s), type and condition of living accommodation, presence/absence of downstairs toilet, ease of access to the home, proximity of neighbours, attendance by home help/public health nurse/private carers, day centre attendance, security of food supply and finance, social activities, contact with close relatives and contingency arrangements for emergency assistance in the case of frailer older people who live alone. Also, transport services need scrutiny. Does the patient drive a car and if so, is the patient likely to be safe/competent? In the case of frail older people, details of community day centre and local respite support to their carers are very important. These details are essential for a complete picture of the older person's home life, social circumstances and level of personal security.

Pearl 8: Physical Examination Must Be Rigorous

For various reasons, older people may not give a complete history or a clear account of their symptoms. Sometimes, older people have so many disorders and complain of so many symptoms that the person taking the history may become muddled and unfocused. This can lead to missed diagnoses, unless the physical examination is rigorous and thorough. Performing high quality and thorough examinations will usually identify the more subtle, but no less important problems that the patient may not articulate when giving the history.

Pearl 9: Structured, Comprehensive Assessment Is Crucially Important

In addition to conventional history and examination in older people, routine assessment of (i) cognition, (ii) gait and balance, (iii) supine and standing blood pressure, (iv) activities of daily living (ADL) function, (v) mood, (vi) vision,
(vii) hearing are essential in all older patients. Without doing these things routinely, common and often easily treatable pathology may be missed.

Pearl 10: Family History Matters

Some students and doctors disregard the older patient's family history as irrelevant and don't enquire about illness patterns in first degree relatives. This is a mistake; family history *is* important in a variety of common (and less common) conditions. Examples include type 2 diabetes mellitus, Alzheimer's disease, hypertension, stroke and colorectal cancer.

Pearl 11: Substance Abuse Happens in Older People too

Abuse of alcohol, hypnotics and so-called 'recreation' drugs occurs in older people as well as in younger people, although not as frequently. Chronic alcohol abuse is under-diagnosed in older people; failure to recognize alcohol dependency in older patients hospitalized with acute illness can have disastrous, irreversible consequences, such as Wernicke's encephalopathy. Equally, many older people take benzodiazepine hypnotics every night, sometimes over a period of decades; abrupt discontinuation of a long-term benzodiazepine (e.g. in a patient hospitalized with acute infection) can result in an acute benzodiazepine withdrawal syndrome manifesting as acute hyperactive delirium. Driving a car whilst under the influence of alcohol can happen quite readily in an older driver, with serious consequences in terms of accident and injury. Older people with dementia may not appreciate risky situations as readily as when they had normal cognition, with resultant misadventure and injury e.g. standing on chairs, climbing step ladders.

Pearl 12: Like Young Children, Older People Require Routine Immunizations

Immunization is highly effective in the older population, particularly in relation to prevention of influenza, pneumococcal infection, herpes zoster and pertussis. Older people should be asked about their recent immunizations, as these may be overlooked or withheld without good clinical grounds.

Tips for the OSCE

(i) Speak slowly and clearly.
(ii) Be prepared for multiple medical conditions and polypharmacy.
(iii) Focus on what is bothering the patient at the present time, avoid devoting too much time to previous medical conditions.
(iv) Be organized and thorough in your physical and cognitive examination.
(v) Blood pressure measurement, fundoscopy, otoscopy and rectal examination are fundamental to the thorough examination of the older person.
(vi) Gait and balance assessment are essential to examination of an older patient, particularly those older people with impaired balance or falls. The 'get-up-and-go' test reveals a great deal: simply instruct the patient to rise from a sitting position, walk 3 metres, turn around and sit down again.

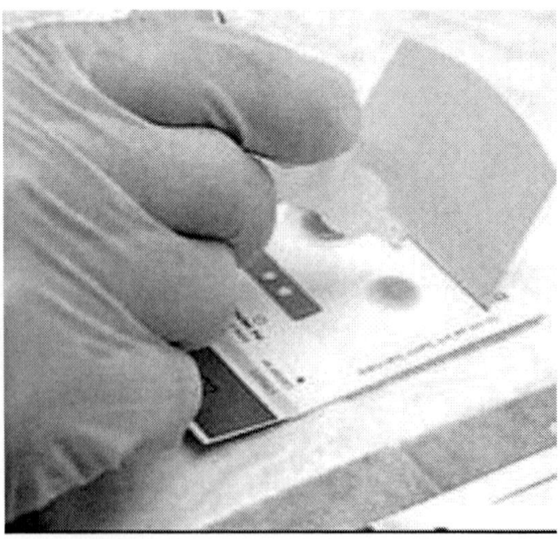

Figure 5. Like the urinalysis test, the FOB test is simple to perform and gives instant, important diagnostic information.

Student Check-list

1. List this older patient's active medical problems in order of priority.
2. Give the details of this older patient's social circumstances and social supports.
3. Assess this older patient's cognitive status.
4. Assess this older patient's functional status in relation to his/her activities of daily living.
5. Assess this older patient's medication in relation to its appropriateness. Are all of his/her medications clearly indicated? Is he/she experiencing actual adverse drug reactions or is he/she at significant risk of adverse drug reactions?
6. Test this stool sample for occult blood. Know the theory behind the faecal occult blood (FOB) test (Figure 5); know how to perform and interpret the FOB test. Remember, 'blue means blood'.

It Happened to me

Mr Smith (not his real name) was a prosperous 76 year old farmer living in central England. He presented to hospital with a two week history of bloody diarrhoea and an estimated 6 kg weight loss over a period of one month. He had a previous history of colonic diverticulitis, hypertension and mild osteoarthritis. He was married, had two sons and remained active in the day-to-day running of the farm. He was taking regular paracetamol and PRN ibuprofen for his arthritis, enalapril for his hypertension and ispaghula husk to prevent constipation. It was presumed that his current weight loss and bloody diarrhoea represented an acute exacerbation of his diverticular disease. On examination, he had a low-grade pyrexia, his abdomen was mildly distended and diffusely tender, and there was easily discernable blood on the glove on rectal examination. A plain film of abdomen showed a diffusely distended colon with multiple areas of mucosal oedema (radiological "thumb-printing" sign positive). Stool cultures were repeatedly negative for common dysenteric pathogens, as well as for ova, cysts and parasites. The patient had not been exposed to antibiotics. The patient proceeded to colonoscopy which showed diffuse colitis with multiple mucosal ulcers and bleeding points. Biopsies were taken and the patient was started on corticosteroids on the presumption of inflammatory bowel disease being the diagnosis. However, his condition deteriorated over the next 24 hours, despite corticosteroid therapy.

Two days after his colonoscopy, I received a phone call from the hospital histopathology laboratory. The pathologist reviewing the patient's colonic biopsy slides informed me that they showed typical features of cytomegalovirus (CMV) colitis; the diagnosis was confirmed later that day with specific virological analysis. CMV colitis being an AIDS-defining illness, the patient was tested for HIV infection and found to be HIV-positive. When the patient's condition had improved with appropriate antiviral therapy, it emerged from more detailed history-taking that his principal risk factor for HIV infection was sporadic, unprotected sex with gay men who frequented a public house near his home.

Lesson 1: Older people sometimes engage in risky sexual behaviour exposing them to risk of HIV infection and other sexually-transmitted infections. All patients, regardless of age or social status, presenting with acute or subacute bloody diarrhoea should be asked about their HIV risk.

Lesson 2: Never assume a diagnosis of inflammatory bowel disease at any age until there is histological confirmation.

> *"Care more for the individual patient than for the special features of the disease. ... Put yourself in his place ... the kindly word, the cheerful greeting, the sympathetic look -- these the patient understands."*
>
> Sir William Osler

Recommended Reading

[1] *ABC of Geriatric Medicine*, N. Cooper, K. Forrest, G. Mulley, eds. Wiley-Blackwell, Chichester, UK, 2009.

[2] *Elderly Care Medicine,* C. Nicholl, K.J. Wilson, S. Webster. Blackwell Publishing Ltd., Oxford, UK, 2007.

[3] *Oxford Handbook of Geriatric Medicine*. L.K. Bowker, J.D. Price, S.C. Smith. Oxford University Press, UK, 2006.

[4] *Measurement Scales used in Elderly Care.* A. Gupta. Radcliffe Publishing, Oxford, UK, 2008.

In: Learning Clinical Skills
Editors: Bridget Maher and Pat Henn

ISBN: 978-1-62100-409-7

Chapter XVI

Introduction to Skin Examination

Benvon Moran and John Bourke

Topic: Cutaneous Vasculitis

Clinical Case

History

A 27-year-old woman presented to the Accident and Emergency Department with a four-day history of a rash affecting the lower limbs and buttocks. It had started on her lower legs and was spreading proximally.

She complained of associated swelling and pain in her ankles and knees. She felt generally unwell and tired. She reported a two-month history of weight loss.

She had had an upper respiratory tract infection two weeks previously which had been treated with penicillin. There was no previous history of dermatological disease and the rest of the review of symptoms was unremarkable.

She had a past medical history of mild asthma and occasionally took inhaled salbutamol. She had not taken any over-the-counter medications recently. She was a non-smoker and drank five units of alcohol per week. There was no family history of note.

Clinical Examination

The patient appeared generally well. She was apyrexial and normotensive. There were discrete, violaceous, non-blanching papules on the feet, legs and thighs, consistent with palpable purpura. There were also some scattered and coalescing haemorrhagic vesicles on her legs (figure 1). She had bilateral ankle oedema and swelling around the knee joints. The remainder of the clinical examination was normal.

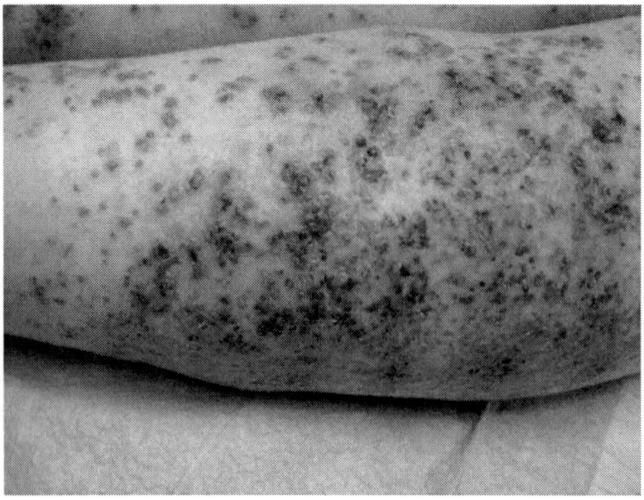

Figure 1. Cutaneous vasculitis

Initial results -Dipstick urinalysis positive for protein and blood.
Diagnosis: Cutaneous vasculitis –unknown cause.

Student Dilemma

1. How do I describe this rash?
2. What other systems should be examined in a patient with a vasculitic rash?
3. What caused this rash?
4. What investigations should be ordered?

Discussion

A methodical approach should be taken when a patient presents with a skin complaint – a complete history and examination should be performed for all patients. The discussion of this clinical case demonstrates the potential complexity of the history and explains how to approach the description of skin lesions.

This patient has a small vessel cutaneous vasculitis. All of the skin should be examined and the morphology of the rash should be described - this will help to formulate differential diagnoses. The table below explains terms for describing individual lesions – colour, shape, surface (eg. scaly), pattern (eg. annular/ring-shaped, dermatomal). Distribution should also be recorded

Cutaneous vasculitis indicates that there is inflammation of the blood vessel walls in the skin. Leakage of blood leads to the purpura seen on examination. Skin biopsy for histological analysis will confirm the diagnosis. Direct immunofluorescence can aid classification of the vasculitis.

Table 1. Morphology

Macule – a flat lesion
Papule – a small, raised lesion (diameter less than 5 mm; figure 2)
Nodule – a large, raised or indurated lesion (diameter greater than 5mm)
Plaque – a raised, flat-topped lesion (figure 3)
Pustule – a yellow, pus-filled papule (figure 4)
Vesicle – a small fluid-filled lesion (diameter less than 5mm; figure 5)
Bulla – a large fluid-filled lesion (diameter greater than 5mm; figure 6)

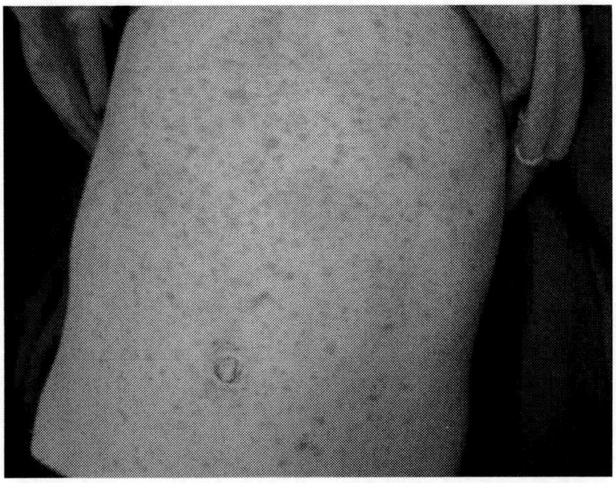

Figure 2. (Papule).

This condition can be self-limiting, but it is very important to examine other systems to ensure that the vasculitis is not affecting other organs which could lead to long-term sequelae (systemic vasculitis). The most important bed-side test to perform in a patient presenting with a vasculitic rash is urinalysis. Haematuria and proteinuria can indicate renal vasculitis which should prompt an urgent nephrology referral. Other organs can also be involved, such as the gastrointestinal tract, which leads to the abdominal symptoms in Henoch-Schonlein purpura. Blood pressure should always be measured in a patient with vasculitis.

In approximately 50% of cases of cutaneous vasculitis, a cause is not identified. The remainder of cases can be attributed to drugs, infection, inflammatory disorders or, rarely, malignancy.

All patients presenting with cutaneous vasculitis should be screened for underlying infection - urine culture, chest x-ray and hepatitis B and C serology should be performed. If the patient is febrile, blood cultures should be taken. A complete drug history should also be recorded. Full blood count, renal and liver function and erythrocyte sedimentation rate (ESR) should be checked.

Anti-nuclear antibodies (ANA), extractable nuclear antigen (ENA), complement levels, anti-neutrophil cytoplasmic antibody (ANCA), cryoglobulins and serum protein electrophoresis should also be measured.

Table 2. Causes of a vasculitic rash

- Infection (eg. β-haemolytic streptococci, viruses)
- Drugs (eg. penicillin, non-steroidal anti-inflammatory drugs)
- Autoimmune disease
  - Systemic lupus erythematosus
  - Rheumatoid arthritis
  - Polyarteritis nodosa
  - Wegener's granulomatosis
- Malignancy (especially haematological)

There are a number of possible causes for this patient's rash. She had had a recent upper respiratory tract infection which could have triggered it (e.g. Henoch-Schonlein purpura). She had penicillin to treat her infection which also could have caused a cutaneous vasculitis. Joint symptoms, weight loss and malaise should prompt investigation into autoimmune causes such as lupus and rheumatoid arthritis. This patient also had haematuria and proteinuria. Urinary protein:creatinine ratio should be measured and a renal ultrasound performed.

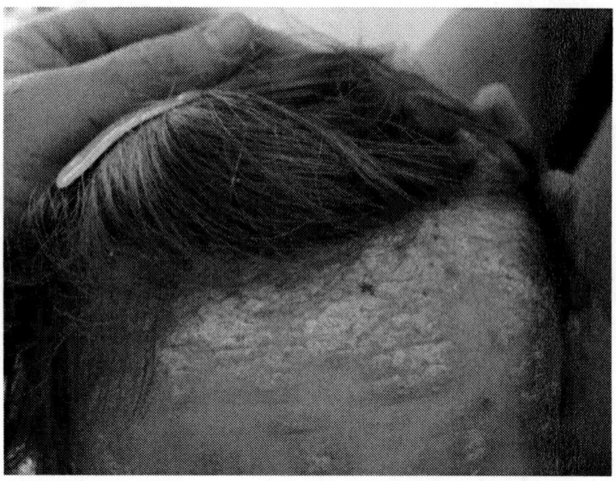

Figure 3. Plaque.

Table 3. Differential diagnosis of a purpuric rash (haemorrhage into the skin)

- Vasculitis
- Vascular disorders
- Senile purpura
- Thrombocytopenia or other coagulation disorder
- Trauma
- Meningococcal disease
- Scurvy

Table 4. Lab spot – Anti-nuclear antibody (ANA)

- Antibody against cell nucleus
- Elevated titres in many autoimmune diseases
  - Lupus
  - Dermatomyositis
  - Sjogren's syndrome
  - Scleroderma
  - Mixed connective tissues disease
  - Rheumatoid arthritis
- Levels increase with
  - Age
  - Drugs (eg. minocycline, biologic agents)
  - Malignancy
  - Females

5% of the normal population will have mildy raised level

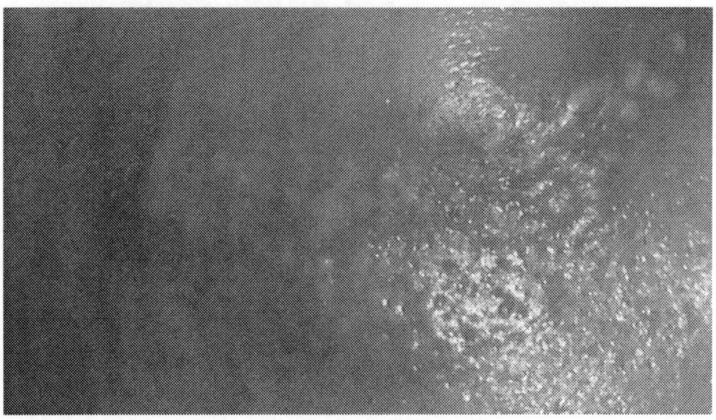

Figure 4. Pustule.

Pitfalls

- Always remember to take a complete drug history – this includes over-the-counter and herbal medications, which patients may forget to mention. Some of these (eg. non-steroidal anti-inflammatory drugs) frequently causes rashes.
- Do not be afraid to look very closely at the rash or lesion you are examining. Some details, such as telangiectasia or a pearly edge, may be more apparent close-up. Explain to the patient that you need to come in closely to examine their skin.
- Do not forget to explain to the patient why a complete skin examination is necessary – understandably they may be confused or upset if they don't know why you're examining their abdomen when the presenting complaint is affecting their face.

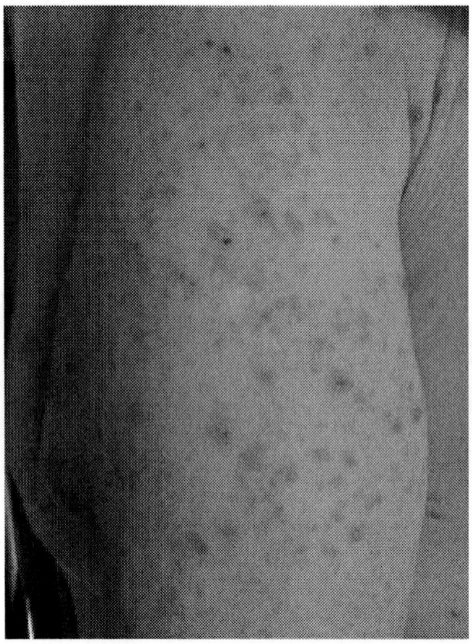

Figure 5. Vesicle.

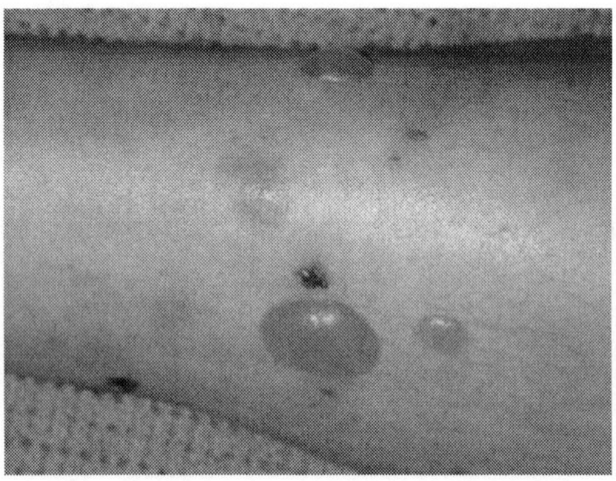

Figure 6. Bullae.

Pearls

- It is as important to touch a rash or lesion as it is to look at it. Determining whether a lesion is flat or raised, smooth or scaly can help to reach the correct diagnosis. You will also need to touch the skin to determine if a rash blanches.
- Complete skin examination includes examination of the hair, nails and mucous membranes. Abnormalities in these areas can help to narrow down the diagnosis (eg. nail pitting and alopecia areata, Wickham's striae on the buccal mucosa and lichen planus). It is also important not to miss 'lesions' in this area in acute dermatoses such as Stevens-Johnson syndrome and toxic epidermal necrolysis. As well as examining the oral mucosa, the eyes, genital and perianal areas need to be examined. If these areas are not examined, permanent corneal scarring can result from eye involvement, or, more acutely, urinary retention from genito-urinary involvement.

- Always offer all patients a chaperone before a full skin examination.
- Ensure that there is adequate light for the examination (natural daylight is preferable). Subtle signs may be missed if the lighting is suboptimal.
- A handtorch or penlight is necessary for examination of the oral mucosa.
- Be aware of the spectrum of normal skin. Be observant when examining patients for other reasons (e.g. listening to the chest) and use it as practice for performing skin examination. Commonly seen benign lesions include naevi, seborrhoeic keratoses, Campbell de Morgan spots and striae.
- Check for palpable lymphadenopathy if a cutaneous malignancy is suspected.

Tips for the OSCE

- At the OSCE you will have a short amount of time to interview or examine the patient with a dermatological complaint. Start with the basics, and it will be possible to gather most of the important information.

History

- *Is the rash itchy*, or otherwise symptomatic? (excoriations are a good clue!).
- Where and when did it start?
- Has anything made it better or worse?

Examination

- Examine the rash, and tell the examiner that you would like to examine all of the skin.
- Describe the rash
  - *Is it scaly?* (describe surface)
  - Morphology (eg. papular, pustular, etc.)
  - Colour (eg. erythematous, violaceous)
  - Distribution

Differential Diagnosis

- Tell the examiner what you think is the most likely diagnosis.
- Also include a number of differential diagnoses if appropriate (if the patient has obvious psoriatic plaques on the elbows, there may not be a need to list other differential diagnoses, but if the patient has a widespread erythematous papular rash, there may be a wide differential diagnosis).

Table 5. Student Check-list

- Describe the cutaneous findings in the clinical case above
- List five causes of purpura
- List five causes of cutaneous vasculitis
- What organs can be affected in Henoch-Schonlein purpura?
- What clinical features can be seen with vitamin C deficiency?

It Happened to me

I was asked to review a middle-aged lady in the clinic with a rash on the lower limbs. It had started about two weeks previously and was getting worse. There was a purpuric rash on the lower limbs, consistent with cutaneous vasculitis. There was no obvious trigger identified. All investigations (including renal function and urinalysis) were normal. The patient felt very well and I reassured her that the rash would most likely settle without treatment. The clinic was busy, and I moved on to the next patient.

I had examined the patient's skin, and was confident with the diagnosis. I had taken a past medical history, and enquired about drug intake. I did not, however, take a social history. The patient returned three days later – the rash was much worse, and her legs were oedematous. She worked long shifts at a supermarket till, and was on her feet for prolonged periods. If this had been elicited during the original history, I would have advised her to remain off work and keep her legs elevated to reduce swelling and aid recovery. This error highlights the importance of taking a full history from all patients. It is important to record a patient's occupation – it can exacerbate, or even cause, many skin diseases.

The value of experience is not in seeing much, but in seeing wisely.

Sir William Osler

Further Reading

Graham-Brown R, Burns T. *Lecture Notes: Dermatology.* 10th ed. Wiley-Blackwell; 2011.

In: Learning Clinical Skills
Editors: Bridget Maher and Pat Henn

ISBN: 978-1-62100-409-7

Chapter XVII

Syncope: Reassure or Refer?

Fionnuala Quigley

Clinical Case 1

A ten year old girl attended her general practitioner accompanied by her mother. She gave a history of two episodes of loss of consciousness. Both episodes occurred in the previous 12 months. The first event happened while she was swimming. She lost consciousness and was taken to the local Emergency Department and was discharged later that day. The second episode happened while she was running in the playground at school. Again, she experienced a short episode of loss of consciousness. Similar to the first episode, she was taken to the Emergency Department and discharged later that day. There were no reports of movement of her limbs, incontinence of urine or tongue/lip biting.

Past Medical History: Apart from these episodes, the girl had been well. She was not taking any medication.

Family History: Two months earlier, her 15 year old sister died suddenly while dancing. No definitive cause of death was found at post-mortem examination and the family are awaiting further results.

Clinical examination: The patient appeared clinically well, pulse was 80/min and regular, blood pressure 100/70. On auscultation of her heart, the heart sounds were normal with no evidence of a murmur. Both femoral pulses were present.

The family and personal history is suggestive of an inherited cardiac condition. Therefore, the patient was referred to a cardiologist with a specific interest in this area.

Investigations: ECG, echocardiogram and ambulatory ECG monitoring were normal. Genetic testing for catecholaminergic polymorphic ventricular tachycardia is positive.

Diagnosis: Syncope secondary to catecholaminergic polymorphic ventricular tachycardia.

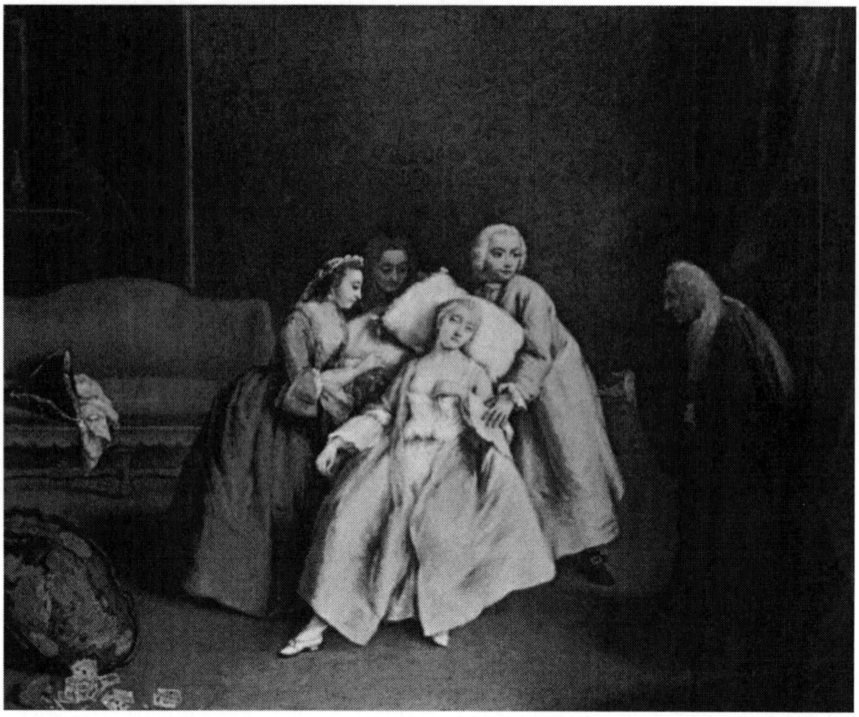

Figure 1. Die Ohnmacht (Fainting). Pietro Longhi. National Gallery of Art.

Clinical Case 2

A general practitioner is called to the home of a 70 year old lady. She was walking in her garden when she was witnessed falling to the ground. Her daughter says her mother lost consciousness for two to three minutes. There was no history of movement of her limbs, incontinence of urine or biting of her lip.

Past Medical History: This was non-contributory. The patient was not taking any medications.

Social History: The patient was a non-smoker and did not drink alcohol. She is a widow living on her own. Her daughter lives next door.

Clinical examination: The patient was alert and orientated. There was a small abrasion on her forehead. She was apyrexial. Pulse rate 88/min. Blood pressure 140/80mmHg supine and 150/85mmHg standing. On auscultation, heart sounds were normal with no audible murmur. Blood glucose 7mmol/l.

The patient was referred to hospital for evaluation. Twenty-four hour ECG monitoring revealed intermittent heart block.

Diagnosis: Syncope secondary to intermittent heart block.

Student Dilemma

- What is meant by syncope?
- What are the potentially relevant points to be elicited in the history in someone presenting with syncope?
- What are the key elements in the clinical examination of a patient with syncope?
- What are the appropriate investigations in a patient with a history of syncope?

Discussion

The presenting complaint in both these cases is syncope, a transient loss of consciousness. It is very important to ascertain what the patient and family mean by a blackout/funny turn as in some instances, they may be describing dizziness or impaired vision. When a patient presents with syncope, a number of differential diagnoses need to be considered:

- Cardiac disease
  - Profound bradycardia
  - Aortic stenosis
  - Hypertrophic Cardiomyopathy
  - Coronary artery anomalies
  - Channelopathies
- Non-cardiac causes
  - Postural hypotension
  - Vasovagal syncope
  - Micturition syncope
  - Hypoglycaemia
  - Hyperventilation
  - Epileptic seizure

Exercise related syncope, in particular, (as reported in Case 1) may suggest an underlying cardiac condition such as Hypertrophic Cardiomyopathy [1], coronary artery anomalies [2], arrhythmogenic right ventricular cardiomyopathy[3], channelopathies [4,5] (congenital long or short QT syndrome, Brugada syndrome, catecholaminergic polymorphic ventricular tachycardia). Family history is key (highlighted in case 1) as certain cardiac conditions such as Hypertrophic Cardiomyopathy [1] and the Channelopathies [4, 5] are genetically determined. Where a cardiac aetiology is suspected, clues may be obtained in the history (Table 1). In these cases, clinical examination needs to focus on pulse rate, blood pressure and heart sounds (Table 2).

In all cases, investigation should commence with blood glucose. If a cardiac cause is suspected, an electrocardiogram, echocardiogram and exercise stress test, and ambulatory ECG monitoring may be done. If a neurological cause is suspected, an EEG and MRI of brain may be appropriate.

Pitfalls

- Always check blood glucose in an unconscious patient. Hypoglycaemia is an easily treatable cause of syncope in a diabetic patient.
- If syncope is exercise–related, consider a cardiac aetiology.

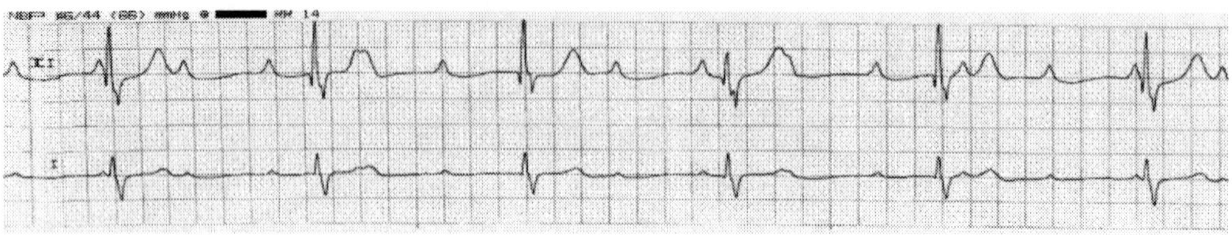

Figure 2. ECG rhythm strip showing third degree heart block.

Table 1. Syncope – clues in the history suggesting cardiac aetiology

- Is syncope exercise related?
- History of palpitations or irregular heart beat?
- History of shortness of breath or fatigue out of proportion to the degree of physical exercise?
- History of exercise related chest pain?
- Family history of sudden unexpected death under the age of 50?

Table 2. Syncope of possible cardiac origin: what to check for on clinical examination (remember that clinical examination may be normal)

- Irregular pulse, bradycardia
- Absent or delayed femoral pulses (coarctation of the aorta)
- Aortic stenosis murmur
- Murmurs associated with Hypertrophic Cardiomyopathy where the murmur intensifies on going from supine to standing position and also increases with the Valsalva manoeuvre

Pearls

- The clue may be in the history. Ask about family history of sudden death under the age of 50, including unexplained road traffic accidents and unexplained drowning while swimming.
- Unexplained syncope in a young athlete in the context of exercise should be considered to be aborted sudden death until proven otherwise [6].

Tips for the OSCE

- Know the differential diagnosis in a case presenting with syncope.
- Take a careful history looking for clues to cardiac aetiology (Table 1).
- Check all pulses including femoral pulses.
- Check blood pressure lying and standing (postural hypotension is a fall in blood pressure > 20/10 from lying to standing).
- Check for a systolic murmur (aortic stenosis and some cases of Hyperptrophic Cardiomyopathy).
- Have a clear plan on how to investigate a patient presenting with syncope.

Student Check List

- What do you look for in the history of a patient with syncope that would direct you to a cardiac cause of syncope?
- What are the most relevant areas in the examination of an individual with a history of syncope?
- What are the appropriate investigations in a patient presenting with syncope?

It Happened to me

An 80 year old lady with known type 2 diabetes came to see me for her routine check- up and for fasting bloods. She reported that she was feeling very well. Her blood pressure was 110/70mmHg, urinalysis showed glycosuria but was otherwise normal. I proceeded to take her bloods including HbA1c, SMAC and serum lipids. A few minutes after taking the blood sample, I turned away to write a prescription. There was a loud bang as the patient suddenly collapsed on the floor. When I reached her, seconds later, she was conscious, complaining of soreness of her wrist. It was immediately clinically apparent that she had sustained a left Colles fracture. The fact that this lady was caring for her ill husband who had COPD made this incident even more upsetting.

Lesson to be learned: Remember the possibility of syncope following phlebotomy. Always consider lying the patient down for a few minutes after the procedure. Every time I see this lady and her moderately deformed wrist, I am reminded of the incident and how it could have been so easily avoided.

He who studies medicine without books sails an uncharted sea, but he who studies medicine without patients does not go to sea at all.

Sir William Osler

References

[1] Maron BJ. Hypertrophic cardiomyopathy:a systematic review. *JAMA* 2002;287:1308-20.

[2] Basso C, Maron BJ, Corrado D,et al. Clinical profile of congenital coronary artery anomalies with origin from the wrong sinus leading to sudden death in young competitive athletes. *J Am Coll Cardiol 2000*;35:1493-501.

[3] Thiene G, Corrado D, Basso C. Arrhythmogenic right ventricular cardiomyopathy/ dysplasia. *Orphanet J Rare Dis* 2007;2:45.

[4] Priori SG, Napolitano C, Tiso N et al. Mutations in the cardiac ryanodine receptor gene (Rryr2) underlie catecholaminergic polymorphic ventricular tachycardia. *Circulation* 2001;103:196-200.

[5] Heidbuchel H, Corrado D, Biffi A et al. Recommendations for participation in leisure time physical activity and competitive sports of patients with arrhythmias and potentially arrhythmogenic conditions. Part 11: ventricular arrhythmias, channelopathies and implantable defibrillators. *Eur J Cardiovasc Prev Rehabil* 2006;13: 676-86.

[6] Firoozi S, Sharma S,McKenna WJ. Risk of competitive sport in young athletes with heart disease. *Heart* 2003;89:710-714.

In: Learning Clinical Skills
Editors: Bridget Maher and Pat Henn

ISBN: 978-1-62100-409-7

Chapter XVIII

Safe for Surgery: Pre-operative Assessment for Anaesthesia and Surgery

Brian O'Donnell

Topic: The Elderly Patient for Hip Fracture Surgery

Clinical Case

A 78 year old lady (Mrs. Browne) was brought by ambulance to the Emergency Department at midday after having fallen in her home. She was found lying on her kitchen floor by neighbours who were concerned for her welfare, as she had not been seen since late the previous day. It was not known how long she had been lying on the floor; however, her previous evening's meal was half eaten on the kitchen table. The Emergency Medical Technicians, who transported her to hospital, reported that she complained of severe pain in her right hip when she was moved. They reported that she was cold to touch and appeared confused and disorientated. She was accompanied to hospital in the ambulance by her daughter.

A collateral history was provided by her daughter. Mrs. Browne lived alone and did not require assistance with activities of daily living. She had a history of hypertension for more than 30 years and was well controlled with bendrofluazide. She had a chest infection three months previously and had developed a chesty cough again in the past week. She was a nonsmoker and took alcohol rarely. She was otherwise in good health. There was no significant family history, and a review of systems was not possible due to Mrs. Browne's acute onset state of confusion.

Clinical examination revealed a non-obese well nourished elderly lady. Temperature 35.5C, blood pressure 102/56, respiratory rate 16/min, pulse 140/min irregularly irregular.

There were no external stigmata of chronic disease. Her skin and oral mucosa appeared dry. At mini-mental state examination she scored 21/30.

Examination of the respiratory system revealed a symmetrically resonant thorax with mild expiratory wheeze bilaterally. Examination of the cardiovascular system revealed a regular tachycardia with audible heart sounds 1 and 2 and no associated murmurs or bruits. Abdominal examination was unremarkable. Examination of the musculoskeletal system revealed a painful, shortened, externally rotated right lower limb with associated oedema and ecchymosis over the greater trochanter.

Initial results revealed elevated white cell count, low haemoglobin, normal platelets, normal coagulation profile, high urea, normal creatinine, normal electrolytes and normal blood sugar (Table 1).

Table 1. Laboratory results

Blood Parameter	Normal Range	Patient's result at presentation
White Cell Count	4-10 x 10^9/L	15 x 10^9/L
Haemoglobin	11.5-16 g/dL	8.2 g/dL
Platelets	150-400 x 10^9/L	325 x 10^9/L
Prothrombin Time	10-14 sec	12 sec
Activated Partial Thromboplastin Time	30-45 sec	37 sec
Urea	2.5-6.7 mmol/L	8.4 mmol/L
Creatinine	70-140 mmol/L	120 mmol/L
Sodium	134-144 mmol/L	138 mmol/L
Potassium	3.5-5.0 mmol/L	3.8 mmol/L
Glucose	3.5-6.5 mmol/l	5.9 mmol/l

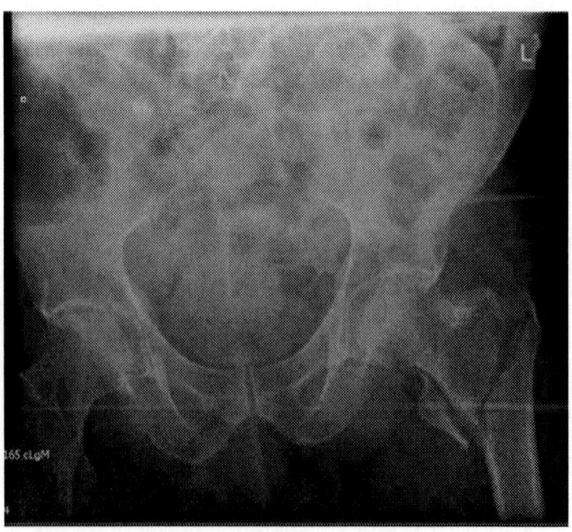

Figure 1. Anteroposterior Radiograph of Pelvis demonstrating an intertrochanteric fracture of the left femur.

A 12 lead ECG revealed sinus tachycardia at a rate of 140 beats per minute. Chest X-Ray was within normal limits. Plain film antero-posterior X-ray views of pelvis revealed an inter-trochanteric hip fracture (Figure 1).

Diagnosis: Inter-trochanteric hip fracture with associated confusional state and abnormal haemodynamic parameters.

Table 2. Student Dilemma

- What is the cause of the tachycardia and hypotension; how is it best treated?
- What is the cause of the patient's acute deterioration in cognitive ability?
- Why is Mrs. Browne anaemic?
- How do I manage this patient's pain prior to corrective hip surgery?

Discussion

Mrs. Browne's case presents three important problems.

1. She has haemodynamic derangement - tachycardia and hypotension. She also has evidence of dehydration (dry mucous membranes and high urea) and a normochromic, normocytic anaemia.
2. She has suffered a common, painful fragility fracture of her hip which will require anaesthesia and surgery. Analgesia prior to and following surgery is a priority.
3. The aetiology of Mrs. Browne's acute confusional state is unclear. It is noteworthy that she lived independently prior to the fall, that she may have been lying on the kitchen floor for a protracted period of time, and that she had mild hypothermia on admission to the Emergency Department.

Hypotension and tachycardia have many possible causes. Blood pressure can be thought of as a product of cardiac output and systemic vascular resistance. Cardiac output is determined by multiple factors which include heart rate, stroke volume and myocardial contractility. Stoke volume, in turn, is reliant upon an adequate circulating blood volume, sufficient diastolic time to permit ventricular filling and adequate contractility to permit forward blood flow. Therefore, hypotension and tachycardia may occur as a result of a reduction in any of the factors which influence cardiac output or systemic vascular resistance. Causes include:

- Hypovolaemia (moderate to severe dehydration, blood loss)
- Impaired cardiac 'pump' function (ischaemia or infarction, cardiomyopathy)
- Impaired systemic vascular resistance
  - Vasodilating drugs (Angiotensin Converting Enzyme inhibitors, Calcium Antagonists, Angiotensin II Receptor Blockers, General Anaesthesia agents [Propofol, Sevoflurane, Isoflurane])
  - Impaired sympathetic outflow (spinal anaesthesia, spinal cord injury)

In the case of an elderly lady who has sustained a hip fracture, occult bleeding occurs which can precipitate a drop in haemoglobin of more than 2g/dl. Therefore, it is probable that Mrs. Browne has hypovolaemia due to acute blood loss associated with her hip fracture. Mrs. Browne was also found on the floor of her kitchen and may have been immobile for a considerable period of time. Without oral fluid intake, she may have a co-existing water deficit or dehydration. A combination of water deficit and hypovolaemia due to blood loss could result in this patient's haemodynamic derangement.

Therapy: Mrs. Browne had an intravenous line placed and was commenced on warmed intravenous fluid therapy to replace a calculated fluid deficit. Blood was taken for cross-match. On commencement of intravenous fluid therapy, Mrs. Browne's heart rate slowed from 140 to 120 beats per minute over the first hour of therapy.

Pain associated with hip fractures is severe and may precipitate a significant stress response in the patient. Movement of the fracture increases pain. The resultant sympathetic response (fight or flight response) results in tachycardia and hypertension. This response may increase myocardial oxygen demand (higher heart rate and contractility) and reduce myocardial oxygen supply (shorter diastolic time and coronary vasoconstriction). Therefore, appropriate analgesia in the Emergency room may improve patient comfort and reduce the tachycardia.

Analgesic Methods

Non-pharmacologic

- Immobilise the fractured hip in a position which the patient feels most comfortable;
- Minimise the number of clinical and nursing interventions which result in fracture movement;
- Minimise the number of transfers of patient from Emergency room examination trolley to inpatient bed;
- Instigate pressure area monitoring;

Pharmacologic

Systemic Analgesia

- Paracetamol has the advantage of having few adverse effects if used within recommended dosing ranges; however, this simple analgesic will have little effect on Mrs. Browne's pain.
- Non-Steroidal Anti-inflammatory Agents (NSIADs) inhibit cyclo-oxygenase pathways and reduce inflammatory mediators which contribute to pain signaling. NSAIDs in the elderly should be used with caution, particularly in Mrs. Browne's case as she has evidence of dehydration and hypoperfusion which may increase the likelihood of adverse renal and gastrointestinal effects. NSAIDs are not appropriate in this particular case.
- Opiates such as morphine, meperidine and oxycodone are potent analgesics which may be used to treat moderate to severe pain. They may be administered either

enterally or parenterally. Adverse effects include respiratory depression with resultant hypoxia, altered mental state, nausea, pruritis, urinary retention and constipation. Elderly patients are most likely to suffer adverse effects. If administered in the appropriate environment with appropriate patient monitoring, opiates may form a useful part of the analgesic pathway.

Regional Analgesia

- The innervation of the extracapsular hip is predominantly derived from the femoral nerve. Femoral nerve blockade with intermediate or long acting local anaesthetic agents will provide effective analgesia with the limb both at rest and on movement. This analgesic technique has the added advantage of not impairing cognitive function. Providing the appropriate dose of local anaesthetic is used, complications such as local anaesthetic systemic toxicity (LAST) can be avoided.

Therapy: In Mrs. Browne's case, a combination of non-pharmacologic methods and femoral nerve block provided excellent analgesia. This resulted in her heart rate dropping from 120 beats per minute to 100 beats per minute.

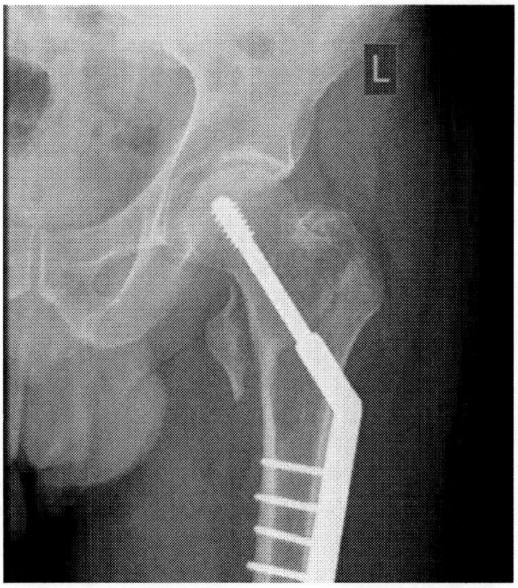

Figure 2. Postoperative Anteroposterior Radiograph revealing a Dynamic Hip Screw internal fixation of left intertrochanteric hip fracture.

Acute Confusional State is common in elderly patients presenting to hospital. Unfamiliar environments, anxiety, pain, dehydration, co-existing infection (pulmonary, urinary tract etc), altered blood glucose and electrolytes, hypothermia, uraemia, myocardial ischaemia and many other problems may contribute to the aetiology of acute confusional states in the elderly patient. Mrs. Browne was cold, dehydrated, hypovolaemic, anaemic and in pain on presentation. After commencement of warmed intravenous fluid therapy and appropriate analgesia, Mrs. Browne became less confused and was able to recount the story of her fall and the subsequent night spent on the kitchen floor.

Mrs. Browne was subsequently scheduled for operative fixation of her hip fracture. Prior to surgery, she received three litres of warmed intravenous Hartman's solution and two units of warmed packed red cells. Her cognitive status returned to normal, as did her haemodynamic parameters. She underwent dynamic hip screw internal fixation of her left hip (Figure 2) under spinal anaesthesia 24 hours following initial presentation.

Lab Spot – Focus on Anaemia

Haemoglobin is essential to oxygen transport around the body. The oxygen carrying capacity of blood is principally determined by haemoglobin concentration (Figure 3). Anaemia may critically reduce tissue oxygen delivery and precipitate cellular hypoxaemia and cell death. The minimal tolerated haemoglobin concentration is dependent upon a number of factors such as age, co-morbidities (ischaemic heart disease, chronic obstructive pulmonary disease etc.) and predicted ongoing blood loss. In Mrs. Browne's case, the presence of anaemia in an elderly lady with hypertension and a predictable ongoing blood loss (from acute fracture and subsequent surgery) were sufficient indications to transfuse packed red cells to increase her oxygen carrying capacity.

- Serum Haemoglobin lower than reference range:
  - Male 13.5-18g/dl
  - Female 11.5-15g/dl
- Identify the red cell profile using mean corpuscular haemoglobin concentration (MCHC) and mean corpuscular volume (MCV)
  - *Normochromic Normocytic*
    - Normal MCHC and MCV
      - Acute blood loss, chronic disease, aplastic anaemia
  - *Normochromic Macrocytic*
    - Normal MCHC and High MCV
      - Pernicious Anaemia (B12 deficiency), folate deficiency, hypothyroidism, alcoholism
  - *Hypochromic Microcytic*
    - Low MCHC and low MCV
      - Chronic blood loss, iron deficiency, thalassaemia, sideroblastic anaemia

Table 3. Equation demonstrating the relationship between haemoglobin concentration and the oxygen carrying capacity of blood

$$\mathbf{CaO_2 = (SaO_2 \times Hb \times 1.34) + 0.003(PaO_2)}$$

CaO_2 = Oxygen Carrying Capacity   Hb = Haemoglobin concentration

SaO_2 = Oxygen Saturation PaO_2= Alveolar Partial Pressure of Oxygen

Pre-operative Assessment

The objectives of the preoperative visit are:

- Meet the patient and develop a doctor patient relationship.
- Perform a full history and clinical examination.
- Identify co-existing pathology and any evident physiologic consequence(s).
- Identify ongoing medical pharmacotherapy and optimize for the perioperative period: e.g. oral hypoglycaemics should be stopped 24 hours prior to surgery, B Blockers should be continued throughout the perioperative period.
- Identify medical conditions which may need to be corrected before surgery: e.g. anaemia may require transfusion; a wheezy chest in a patient with asthma might require bronchodilator therapy.
- Ensure the appropriate fasting interval for solids and fluid have been adhered to (six hours fasting for solids, clear fluids may be taken up to two hours before anaesthesia).
- Review the results of appropriate, targeted preoperative investigations. Order and review further investigations as indicated.
- Inform the patient as to their individualised plan for anaesthesia.
- Obtain consent for anaesthesia and any anaesthesia related procedures.

Pitfalls

- Occult underlying co-morbidities may be present in the apparently ‘fit and healthy’ person presenting for anaesthesia and surgery; therefore it is important to always take a complete history and perform a targeted clinical examination.
- Reliance on ‘routine’ preoperative blood tests, radiology and electrocardiography to exclude significant disease is ill-advised and an expensive waste of resources. Targeted investigations based upon appropriate history taking and physical examination is recommended.

Table 4. American Society of Anesthesiologists (ASA) Classification of Physical Status

ASA I	No underlying disease
ASA II	Underlying systemic disease with minimal or no physical impairment
ASAIII	Underlying systemic disease with significant physical impairment
ASA IV	Life-threatening intercurrent illness
ASA V	Severe life-threatening illness in a moribund patient not expected to survive without surgery
Add the suffix (E) for emergency surgery.	

The American Society of Anesthesiologists Classification of Physical Status scoring system is commonly used by anaesthetists worldwide to group patients based on physical status.

Pearls

- Approach the patient in a calm, friendly, assured manner.
- Patients are normally equally anxious about not waking up from anaesthesia, or worse, waking during surgery, as they are about surgery itself. A confident assuring manner will aid in allaying anaesthesia-related anxieties.
- Always ask about any alternative medicines that the patient may be taking. Even common health supplements can cause interactions with anaesthetic dugs and have been shown to have an adverse impact on factors such a platelet function and surgical blood loss.
- Beware the elderly patient with a systolic murmur in the aortic area! Aortic stenosis can severely compromise myocardial perfusion during anaesthesia and should be sought by clinical examination.
- 'Fitness' for anaesthesia and surgery may be determined by objective assessment of cardiac and pulmonary function (echocardiography, stress echocardiography, lung function tests and cardiopulmonary exercise tests [CPET]). Alternatively, simply asking whether a patient can climb two flights of stairs without becoming breathless or having chest pain has been shown to equate to a physiological status of 'fit for surgery'.

Tips for the OSCE

- Approach the patient in a friendly, considerate and confident manner.
- Take an appropriate targeted history and perform the relevant clinical examination.
- Order and interpret targeted investigations.
- Be prepared to discuss the physiologic relevance of abnormal blood tests, radiology or other investigations, and the management of such abnormalities in the peri-operative period. Don't be afraid to use basic science or 'first principles' in problem solving.

Student Checklist

- Identify the patient, the type and site/side of surgery planned and the indication for surgery.
- Take a complete history and perform targeted physical examination, order appropriate laboratory, radiology and other investigations.

- Identify co-existing morbidities.
- Identify unidentified underlying illness.

The pre-operative assessment should include:

- Full history and clinical examination.
- Targeted laboratory and other relevant investigations.
- Identify correctable, undertreated or new medical conditions.
- Commence appropriate therapy prior to anaesthesia and surgery.
- Monitor objectively patient response to therapy.
- Proceed with anaesthesia and surgery once the desired response has been obtained and the patient has been 'optimised' for surgery.

It Happened to me

An 82 year old male farmer was crushed by a cow and pinned between the cow and a wall. He sustained an intracapsular fracture of his right neck of femur and a subcapital fracture of his right humerus. On arrival at the hospital, he was alert and orientated and in obvious pain. He had no significant medical history, no allergies and took no medicines. Review of systems and clinical examination of respiratory, cardiovascular, abdominal and genitourinary systems was unremarkable. It was noted that the man's haemoglobin was 7 g/dl. The gentleman was administered intravenous fluid therapy, and analgesia was commenced using an intravenous morphine patient controlled analgesia (PCA) device. He was scheduled for urgent surgery later that same day. He did not receive red cell transfusion prior to surgery.

Mid-way through surgery under general anaesthesia, the patient became profoundly hypotensive and tachycardiac with evidence of myocardial ischaemia (ST segment depression on ECG). The surgery was interrupted and the man was rushed to the interventional cardiology suite for emergency angiography following consultation with cardiology. At angiography, he was found to have semi-occlusive lesions in his mid right coronary artery and left sided circumflex artery. Angioplasty resulted in restoration of ST segment toward baseline and intra-coronary stents were placed. The man was transfused with packed red cells and was cared for in the Intensive Care Unit for 48 hours. He underwent completion of surgery on day three of his admission.

Occult vasoocclusive coronary artery disease may be present in elderly patients. Impaired oxygen carrying capacity caused by anaemia due to acute post-traumatic blood loss, combined with the stress response associated with pain and injury, unmasked the asymptomatic coronary artery disease in this man's case. Vigilance and an understanding of the pathophysiology involved prompted early intervention, definitive treatment and a good patient outcome.

The good physician treats the disease; the great physician treats the patient who has the disease

Sir William Osler

Further Reading

Beaudoin FL, Nagdev A, Merchant RC, Becker BM. Ultrasound-guided femoral nerve blocks in elderly patients with hip fractures. *Am J Emerg Med* 2010;28:76-81.

Biccard BM. Relationship between the inability to climb two flights of stairs and outcome after major non-cardiac surgery. *Anaesthesia* 2005;60:588-93.

British Orthopaedic Association and British Geriatric Society. *The Care of Patients with Fragility Fracture Accessed April 30th 2011.* Available at: http://www.fractures.com/pdf/BOA-BGS-Blue-Book.pdf.

Garcia-Miguel FJ, Serrano-Aguilar PG Lopez-Bastida J. Preoperative assessment. *Lancet* 2003;362:1749-57.

Hill S, Carless PA, Henry DA, Carson JL, Hebert PPC, Henderson KM, McClelland B. *Transfusion thresholds and other strategies for guiding allogenic red blood cell transfusion.* Cochrane Database of Systematic Reviews 2000; 1:CD002042.k.

Kaye AD, Kucera I, Sabar R. Perioperative anaesthesia clinical considerations of alternative medicines. *Anesthesiol Clin North America* 2004;22:125-39.

Smith GH, Tsang J, Molyneux SG, White TO. The hidden blood loss after hip fracture. *Injury* 2011; 42: 133-5.

In: Learning Clinical Skills
Editors: Bridget Maher and Pat Henn
ISBN: 978-1-62100-409-7

Chapter XIX

The Psychiatric Interview and Mental State Examination

Aisling Campbell

Case History

A 60 year old woman presented with a ten week history of "anxiety", characterised by anxious ruminating about her behaviour towards family members in the past. She was preoccupied with a belief that she had mistreated a brother who had subsequently died. On examination, she was vague as to the details of this event but expressed the belief that she was a bad person and that her current presentation was due to "childishness". She denied feeling depressed. A collateral history, however, revealed that she had a previous history of several similar episodes of anxious ruminations which would commence for no obvious external reason and generally lasted for three to four months at a time, and were associated with poor sleep, decreased self care and poor appetite. It was clear that the presentation and previous history were consistent with a mood disorder and were atypical of a straightforward anxiety disorder. A diagnosis of recurrent depressive disorder was made. The patient had a good response to antidepressant medication and described herself as having been "in a black hole" prior to treatment.

Discussion

This case illustrates how, what at face value appeared to be an anxiety disorder, proved in fact to be a depressive illness with obsessional ruminations which were secondary. The patient herself was a poor historian and did not give a clear history of depressed mood. However, close examination of her symptoms and of the psychopathology as well as of the onset and course of her illness from collateral history, suggested that a recurrent depressive disorder was the most likely diagnosis. Treatment of this patient as simply suffering from an anxiety disorder would have been unsuccessful and potentially dangerous, as patients with depressive disorders have a significant risk of suicide.

The Importance of History-taking Skills in Psychiatry

Psychiatry could be considered the medical specialty in which clinical skills are most vital, as psychiatric diagnosis relies almost entirely on the history-taking and mental state examination skills of the psychiatrist. While many psychiatric syndromes have organic causes (and there is an ever-growing body of evidence for neurochemical correlates of numerous psychiatric disorders), there is still no armamentarium of laboratory tests or measurements that support psychiatric diagnoses robustly. In this specialty, more than any other, the clinician is on his own. This may be seen as a disadvantage – indeed psychiatry is often incorrectly accused of being unscientific for these reasons – but it is in reality an advantage. Psychiatry hones clinical interview skills: the psychiatrist must be a strategist and tactician, using wiliness and charm in order to gain meaningful information so as to reach an unbiased diagnosis. There is no more satisfying experience in medicine than to establish and defend a psychiatric diagnosis on the basis of detailed, thorough historical information and psychopathology that has been forensically teased out.

The psychiatrist in search of a diagnosis may be compared to the detective interviewing a possible suspect – he may well know that he has his quarry in his sights (paradoxically, an experienced psychiatrist can often make a diagnosis in three minutes) but he must carefully collect his information and construct his evidence so that it is robust and defensible in the face of scrutiny.

Psychiatric diagnosis is based largely on establishing the existence of a cluster of symptoms and psychopathology and the diagnostic process must therefore be particularly rigorous. However, while psychiatric interviewing must be forensic in its attention to detail, it must also be empathic and respectful of the patient. A good psychiatrist can establish and maintain a therapeutic and supportive relationship with the patient, while being ruthless in sifting through the clinical information to reach the correct diagnosis; he establishes the specifics and particularities of the patient's case, while never losing sight of the generalities.

A thorough psychiatric interview, particularly one that includes extensive questioning on personal history, can be therapeutic in itself. The initial interview with a patient is often the most memorable one – the psychiatrist who has been fortunate enough to interview the patient first may gain the most in-depth understanding of the patient and his illness.

The old saw of the "biopsychosocial model" is often regurgitated by students in oral examinations (no doubt it is perceived by students as provoking a reflex response in some examiners): the reality is that the psychiatrist is uniquely placed to bring a multitude of perspectives on a patient's case, not only a biomedical perspective, but also a knowledge of psychological factors and cultural factors and to weave these together to produce a meaningful formulation. While other members of the psychiatric multidisciplinary team will bring their own specific expertise to a case, psychiatric diagnosis should be the central focus, as management plans, risk assessment and prognosis are all diagnosis-dependent. Accurate psychiatric diagnosis throws all other issues into relief and brings clarity to clinical practice.

The purposes of the psychiatric interview are to establish diagnosis, elucidate the biological, psychological and social factors that bear on the patient's problems, and to develop the therapeutic alliance.

The Psychiatric Interview: Context

The approach to the psychiatric interview is context-dependent. A different approach will be required by a general practitioner who suspects that a patient's physical complaints mask an underlying psychiatric disorder, vis-a-vis the approach used by the psychiatrist interviewing a manic patient who requires involuntary admission. Likewise, the liaison psychiatrist interviewing a patient with pseudo-seizures who has been discharged from medical care will use a different approach from the psychiatrist who is assessing for medicolegal purposes. The influence of different contexts on the approach is somewhat beyond the scope of this chapter, but it must be acknowledged that, in real life, many patients with psychiatric disorders present for treatment at best reluctantly. While patients will usually voluntarily seek treatment for, say, chest pain or acute dyspnoea, many patients with psychiatric disorders lack insight. The patient's subjective account of his presenting complaint, therefore, may bear little relation to the actual diagnosis. Another problem is that much of the terminology used in psychiatry has a colloquial usage also. For instance, many patients describe themselves as being "depressed" but are not suffering from a depressive disorder. The clinician must therefore be suspicious and must not take presenting complaints at face value. Taking a psychiatric history involves following a range of symptoms down many blind alleys, in an effort to elucidate the patient's subjective experience and to establish the exact nature of psychopathology from the patient's description.

Teasing out the Symptoms

In history-taking, the symptoms must be teased out, with a range of differential diagnoses being considered, tested and discarded or retained. It is helpful – indeed essential – to use a diagnostic hierarchy. Organic disorders must be considered first, followed by major psychoses and affective disorders. Only once these have been ruled out can neurotic disorders be considered. Simultaneously, personality disorders and substance misuse must be considered as possible comorbid disorders. This approach helps to direct and focus the psychiatrist's questioning, and ensures that serious psychiatric disorders will not be missed. There is no safety net of laboratory tests to protect the psychiatrist who has made an incorrect diagnosis. The vignette below provides further illustration:

A 22 year old student was referred by his general practitioner for treatment of panic disorder. He had become agitated over the previous few months and his family had been concerned about his friendship with a much older man. The week before referral, he had suddenly travelled by plane to London, without warning his family, and remained there, sleeping rough, until he was found by a family member and taken home. At interview, he was unable to explain his actions but presented as vague and unforthcoming. He denied psychotic symptoms but when his mother was brought into the interview to provide collateral information, she asked the patient if he had mentioned that on the way to clinic he had been concerned that a road sign indicating "Danger" had referred to him. Further interviewing revealed paranoid ideation and hallucinations, and a diagnosis of schizophreniform psychosis was made. He was successfully treated with antipsychotic medication.

This case shows the importance of utilising the diagnostic hierarchy to provide a safeguard against error. Symptoms do not a diagnosis make. In the case illustrated above, assuming that the diagnosis is that of panic disorder, simply because the patient describes panic (a nonspecific symptom which in itself is virtually useless in reaching a diagnosis), will lead to a far more serious disorder – schizophrenia – being missed. As the treatment of schizophrenia is entirely different from that of panic disorder, at best this would result in appropriate treatment being delayed and at worst, it could lead to a significant risk of suicide (far commoner in schizophrenia than in panic disorder).

In taking a psychiatric history, the physician must therefore hold in his mind the diagnostic hierarchy, and must, in the context of the patient's answers, constantly test various diagnostic hypotheses against this hierarchy. At the same time, he must be aware of the impact of mental state and lack of insight on the information provided by the patient, and must maintain a therapeutic relationship as far as possible. Quite a tall order! A structured approach to history-taking is a great help in this context, but it must be remembered that patients have not read text-books and may not give answers in the order in which the doctor desires them. The trainee or student may find that jotting down headings such as those outlined below will help in "editing" the information later for the purposes of case presentation. Patients will tend to discuss those issues foremost in their minds first; this may be abuse that the patient suffered many years ago, for example, rather than their current depressive symptoms. Part of the art of medicine is giving the patient's concerns the attention they deserve while not being swayed from formulating a differential diagnosis. A patient who lacks insight will present a particular challenge in this regard; a patient who, for example, believes himself to be under the control of an alien force is unlikely to have much patience with the doctor whose main interest is in establishing that this is a first-rank symptom of schizophrenia. The wily doctor will acknowledge the very real anxieties of such a patient while continuing to explore and establish the details of history and psychopathology, on the sly as it were. Basic curiosity about human beings should not be underestimated as a core attribute of the skilled psychiatrist – the more the psychiatrist knows about his patient, the symptoms, their precipitants and the rest of his patient's life experience, the more precisely he can assess, manage and prognosticate.

Pearls and Pitfalls

- Psychiatric interviews may occur in a range of contexts, each requiring a specific approach.
- Symptoms should not be taken at face value and must be explored in detail.
- The diagnostic hierarchy should be borne in mind, as should comorbidity.

Beginning the Psychiatric Interview

As in all branches of medicine, the context will set the tone of the interview. The approach will be different with a patient who is presenting semi-electively with a several month history of eating disorder, compared with the approach used with a manic patient in the Accident & Emergency Department. However, it should be acknowledged that there are very few elective presentations in psychiatry. Most psychiatric disorders are distressing and patients usually benefit from a reassuring manner. Some patients will be reluctant attendees – especially those who lack insight – and this must be anticipated by the doctor. The usual niceties should apply – doctors and medical students should introduce themselves; shaking hands is not obligatory. Some doctors may feel that shaking hands puts the patient at ease – the experience of the writer is that a handshake is not necessary in this regard and may create a false sense of friendliness which may not be sustainable throughout the consultation. However, interviewing and history-taking involve a degree of acting – and each doctor must find his own personal style. Patients quickly pick up if the doctor is tense himself, or is being false.

The doctor should clarify the purpose of the consultation, and the referral source if appropriate, as well as his own role. It is often useful to advise the patient roughly what sort of questions will be asked, how long the interview is likely to take (it is a source of constant amazement to this author how many patients believe a psychiatric assessment can be completed in ten minutes when in reality it should take from 50 minutes to 90 minutes). Depending on context, it may be wise to advise the patient that particular questions will be asked – for example, patients attending for elective medicolegal assessment should be advised clearly that family and personal history will be explored – they rarely expect this and may object if not alerted to it beforehand.

Patients should be advised that the interviewer may take notes during the consultation. Although many patients are uncomfortable with note-taking, in real-life clinical practice there is rarely time to write up notes afterwards. Reassurances should be given to the patient regarding the confidentiality of such notes, and medical students should clarify that notes will be anonymised and destroyed afterwards.

While the standard advice with regard to interviewing is to start with open, non-leading questions as far as possible, the degree to which the doctor controls the interview or otherwise will depend on the patient's degree of spontaneity and focus. A very depressed patient may well be unspontaneous and monosyllabic and may require some fairly closed questions; likewise a manic, or even a circumstantial patient may require the interviewer to take a significant degree of control of the interview. The approach required will generally be obvious in the first five minutes.

History of Presenting Complaint

Before launching into the history of the patient's presenting complaint, basic information such as date of birth, occupation and other similar details should be requested. This may already have been obtained by administrative staff but such basic questioning can help to put the patient at ease. The doctor will then ask the patient to describe what has been going wrong recently. As described above, the patient may not necessarily give his story in the order preferred by the doctor. In this case, it is best to allow the patient to speak for a minute before tactfully moving him on to the presenting complaint. For example:

Doctor: "Tell me what has been going wrong for you lately".

Patient: "I think I've been depressed all my life really. As far back as when I was three or four, I remember being really unhappy. I've taken five overdoses in my life, and my problems got worse five years ago when my husband went to prison. And now I'm worried about my son too, he's getting in with the wrong crowd."

Doctor: "It sounds as though there really have been a lot of serious difficulties for you over the years. I would like to explore all of the things you mention in detail, in a few minutes. Right now I would really like to focus on the symptoms you've been having very recently so that we can choose the right treatment for you."

This interview could clearly go in many directions – the patient's previous overdoses, her unhappy childhood – but the doctor has kept the focus on current symptomatology in a tactful way, while remaining empathic. Patients usually do not appreciate the importance of diagnostic accuracy, and medical students and trainees in psychiatry often get side-tracked by other issues raised by the patient and fail to explore the psychopathology in detail.

The doctor must explore in detail the nature of the current symptoms, the onset, time course of same, and any precipitating factors. He must then explore in detail any associated symptoms including ones that may not have been mentioned by the patient. For example, if the patient complains of depression, the doctor must establish first of all that the patient really does have low mood (and not some other problem such as anxiety) and then explore sleep disturbance, concentration, appetite disturbance, diurnal variation in mood and so on.

As with all medical history-taking, the interview should begin with open questions and progress gradually to closed ones, and all questions should be non-leading. Anxious patients in particular, are likely to give the doctor the answers they think he wants so the question "You're not waking early in the morning, are you?" is likely to be followed by an answer in the negative, and the doctor will be none the wiser. However, with vague historians especially, it may be necessary to focus on specific detail in a closed-questioning manner, as illustrated in the example below:

Doctor: "You've told me that you believe you are suffering from depression. Can you try to describe what this feels like?"

Patient: "Well, you're the doctor, you should know about depression."

Doctor: " Yes, I do know about depression, but I'm interested in what you yourself are experiencing. Perhaps you could try to paint a picture in words of what you feel?"

Patient: "Well, you know, I'm down-and-out kind of thing."

Doctor: "What do you mean by down-and-out?"

Patient: "Well, it's kind of like couldn't be bothered. No energy. You know what I mean."

Doctor: "When you say you couldn't be bothered, does that affect how you manage to do things at home and at work" [here the doctor is "fishing" while trying not to be leading].

Patient: "Yeah, you know I just don't have the interest any more. I go through the motions but my heart isn't in it. And I think I'm paranoid, I don't answer the phone to my friends, and I've been isolating myself."

Here, the patient, while describing an apparently genuinely depressed affect, throws in another possible symptom – being "paranoid" – which must be followed up by the doctor. However, the likelihood is that the patient is simply describing the social withdrawal that is common in depression, and is not psychotic. The doctor here should focus on establishing the core mood, explore related symptoms such as sleep and concentration, and then return to the question of paranoid ideation.

It is essential that the doctor be alert to these additional symptoms and cues that may arise in the interview. Some will prove to be red herrings but some may be of vital importance as in the example below:

Doctor: "Can you tell me why your GP referred you for assessment here in the hospital?"

Patient: I don't know, there's nothing wrong with me as you can see. Can I go now?"

Doctor: "I'd like to ask you a few more questions before we decide what's best for you. It sounds like your GP was worried about you if he sent you here today straight after seeing you."

Patient: "I'm absolutely fine Doc, the spirit is in me and I feel good. I don't want to waste your time."

[Here the phrase "the spirit is in me" is unusual and should alert the doctor to the possibility the patient may have a psychotic illness. However, such comments may be missed if the doctor is impatient and is not listening.]

Doctor (missing the unusual phrase)*: "No, it's really important that you stay. Now, why did you go to see your GP today?"*

Patient: "It was my parents, they called my GP but I didn't want to see him. Gabriel came and he made me feel unhappy because he gets into my brain."

[It sounds here as though the patient is having some sort of psychotic experience. However, if the doctor is not alert to this possibility he will miss the opportunity to ask about "Gabriel" and this opportunity may not return.]

Doctor (again missing the unusual content of the patient's conversation): *"I'm just interested in what the GP thought was wrong with you. What did your parents tell him?"*

Imagine how the interview might have progressed if the doctor had picked up the cues indicated above.

Patient: "It was my parents, they called my GP but I didn't want to see him. Gabriel came and he made me feel unhappy because he gets into my brain."

Doctor: "Who is Gabriel – how does he get into your brain?" [Strictly speaking, there are two questions here – not the ideal approach, but the doctor is appropriately eager to capture what may be crucial psychopathology and the moment may pass all too soon. In this situation a double question is justifiable.]

Patient: "Have you never heard of the Angel Gabriel? He comes to me and all the spirits in me suddenly go quiet because he is very big and covers my brain so I can't think."

There are two crucial areas that the doctor must pursue in this instance – the patient is indicating that the angel Gabriel in some way controls him, possibly his thinking, so thought passivity delusions must be explored in detail. Furthermore, the patient refers to the spirits in him "going quiet" suggesting that he may be hallucinating voices or sounds that he perceives as coming from spirits. Again, this must be explored in detail. Through a combination of luck and the patient's preoccupations, the doctor may well eventually arrive at the correct diagnosis but this is no substitute for intelligent and thorough interviewing technique. This is particularly important – as shown in this example – where the patient is psychotic. Lack of insight is common in psychotic disorders and will prevent a patient from fully cooperating with the doctor's wish to make an accurate diagnosis. In the example given, the patient does not believe that he is ill, but rather that the angel Gabriel is controlling his mind – from the medical perspective the two are the same, but to the patient, he has a problem which cannot be solved by modern medicine! Psychiatric interviewing differs therefore from medical history-taking in that patients may not form the usual alliance with the doctor in order to find out the cause of their symptoms – patients with chest pain, for instance, generally want it investigated and treated. Insight tends to be lacking in psychotic disorders, in the context of elated mood because the patient may have an inflated sense of well-being and in disorders which involve an addictive component such as alcoholism or eating disorders (where denial is a key feature).

From the patient's point-of-view, it is important that the doctor listens to what he has to say and demonstrates a genuine interest. A logical series of questions from the interviewer goes a long way in this regard. By the same token, an interviewer who seems at a loss for the next question gives the impression of being unempathic, as in the following example. Ultimately, lack of empathy is likely to affect the therapeutic relationship.

Patient: "Yes, my OCD (obsessive-compulsive disorder) has been bad for the past five years but it got really bad about ten months ago."

Doctor: "What sort of rituals have you been doing?"

Patient: "Well, the usual things, you know, I have to wash my hands about twenty times after using the toilets. And touching things, you know. But it's really bad in the last ten months."

Doctor: "What happened ten months ago?"

Patient: "That was when our son died from meningitis."

Doctor: "Yes, well, and how has your sleep been?"

Patient (looking nonplussed)*: "Oh, it's been fine."*

Awkward silence.

In this example, an inexperienced doctor has forgotten the next question – he is so preoccupied with trying to think of what to ask, that he is unable to respond empathically to the patient. It should be obvious that this type of mistake does not foster a working therapeutic relationship, and at best will annoy the patient who is then less likely to cooperate. There is a certain amount of acting involved in interaction with patients – over the years this becomes second nature, to the degree that, even on a bad day, the doctor will come across as empathic. This only comes with practice.

A detailed description of all the different types of psychopathology is beyond the scope of this chapter but suffice to say that the doctor must clearly establish beyond reasonable doubt that the patient has sufficient psychopathology to support the differential diagnosis, and must ensure that important disorders high in the diagnostic hierarchy have been carefully considered. The commonest error made by inexperienced students and trainees is a failure to adequately focus on psychopathology in detail, thereby leading to diagnosis which is based on insufficient information and invalid deductions. The detail obtained must allow the doctor to not only make an accurate diagnosis, but also to have a full understanding of the patient's experiences, the duration and course of the symptoms and the possible risks associated with the patient's symptoms. The doctor should establish what treatments the patient has already tried, and what degree of disability has resulted from the symptoms.

Pearls and Pitfalls

- Explain the purpose and nature of the psychiatric interview at the start.
- Begin with open questions and follow up with closed questions.
- Inadequate attention to the details of the presenting complaint is the commonest error made by inexperienced interviewers.

Previous Psychiatric History

It is logical to follow on from taking a detailed history of the presenting complaint to obtaining a detailed history of previous similar episodes or other psychiatric history. Patients are more likely to cooperate when they see a logical flow to the doctor's questions. It is essential to obtain detailed information on a patient's previous psychiatric history as this will support the differential diagnosis, and inform management including risk management.

It is helpful to introduce the topic by asking the patient – after exploring the presenting complaint – "have you ever had similar symptoms before?" or "have you ever had a similar episode before?" Asking simply if the patient has ever attended a psychiatrist before may lead to a false negative answer as the patient may well have been symptomatic previously but didn't seek treatment or perhaps attended another type of health professional.

If there has been a previous episode, this should be explored in detail – the nature of the symptoms, any treatment received and response to same and particularly any previous suicide attempts (even if the patient has not made a recent attempt or is not currently expressing any suicidal ideation). A previous suicide attempt made with apparently serious intent, or a suicide attempt involving a violent method, significantly increases the lifetime risk of completed suicide. Failure to identify an earlier serious suicide attempt will therefore give the doctor a false impression of the patient's current and future risk. Previous suicide attempts should therefore be asked about specifically – it should not be assumed that the patient will automatically mention them.

Many patients encountered within the psychiatric services have a long history of mental illness and it may be impossible to tease out the detail of numerous previous episodes of illness. In this situation, the student should ask about the patient's first episode, and most recent episode, and should try to establish the pattern over the years. It may be expedient to ask if the patient has had an episode roughly every year, or every two years and so on. An attempt should be made to establish the type of psychopathology involved in these episodes – if it has been the same as current psychopathology, or has been significantly different. With complex disorders such as bipolar affective disorder, it is essential to tease out the various treatments that have been tried and when, and the response to each treatment. Ultimately, this can only be done accurately by obtaining previous medical records and a collateral history, but these may not be available immediately and treatment decisions may need to be made urgently.

Many patients with chronic psychotic illnesses have minimal insight and may give inaccurate histories. In this case, it is worth asking the patient directly if he was ever treated with different antipsychotics (giving trade names) as the patient may not spontaneously proffer this information. Likewise, asking about a "monthly injection" (depot antipsychotic) may yield results. Where an affective disorder is suspected, it is essential to ask about periods of elated mood. Because elated mood is usually not subjectively distressing, patients may not recall these periods when discussing past history. However, some patients with emotionally unstable personality disorder seek a diagnosis of bipolar mood disorder and may inaccurately describe periods of elated mood which, on detailed questioning, turn out to be simply brief fluctuations in mood rather than the true, prolonged elated mood of bipolar disorder. Again, a collateral history is invaluable but may not always be available. Asking specifically about treatment with lithium, or about "electrical treatment" (electro-convulsive therapy) is important where a mood disorder is suspected.

It is essential to obtain a detailed history of past and current alcohol and substance use. Patients who have a history of substance misuse tend to minimise both the amount and the impact of same. When current alcohol abuse is suspected, for instance, pitching the questioning "high" may yield a more honest answer. The following example illustrates the pitfalls of naivety in this situation:

Doctor: Have you been drinking much lately?

Patient: Ah, not really, you know, social drinking.

Doctor: (writing in notes "social drinker") *So, what would that be, a few pints at weekends?*

Patient: (relieved that the doctor seems ready to abandon this uncomfortable line of questioning) *Yeah, a few pints maybe on a Saturday with the lads. You know, we all like our pint. But I'd never drink if I had to work the next day.*

Doctor: OK, and you don't take any street drugs do you?

*Patient: (*again, relieved that his regular cannabis intake is not going to be rigorously pursued*). Well, the odd bit of weed but just once in a while.*

Contrast this with a more suspicious interviewer:

Doctor: Have you been drinking much lately.

Patient: Ah, not really, you know, social drinking.

Doctor: So, what would a typical week's drinking involve?

Patient: Well, I might go out at the weekend with the lads. You know, a few pints.

Doctor: So, if you were out on a Friday night, what would you have? Maybe 20 pints or so and a naggin or two if you went on to a club? (asked in a tone that suggests this is a completely normal drinking).

Patient: Oh, God, not 20 pints, no, maybe more like 12 or 13 and then a few shorts.

Doctor: And maybe a bottle of wine before you'd go out?

Patient: Well, yeah, if it was a big night out.

Doctor: And what about Saturday night? Same again?

Patient: Yeah, probably.

Doctor: And on a Sunday? Would you have the same again?(again, without any hint of his inner shock at the amount the patient is drinking).

Patient: Ah no, I'd cut it down on a Sunday, maybe 7 or 8 pints.

Doctor: And then during the week, what would you do?

Patient (side-stepping the issue) *Oh, I don't go out during the week.*

Doctor: So,would you get a few cans in on week nights?

Patient: Yeah, maybe a few cans.

Doctor: So how many cans would you have at home each night, maybe a couple of six packs?

Although it can be somewhat laborious, extracting accurate information requires a painstaking and tactical approach. The doctor must give the patient the impression that he will not be shocked by any answer and that he considers what is, in reality, a very high level of alcohol intake, to be within the range of normal social drinking. Once the information is given, the doctor can then advise the patient that his drinking is excessive, but this card must not be played too early, or the patient will succeed in minimising his drinking. The same approach may be used for all forms of substance misuse. If the patient has a long history of substance misuse, any previous history of addiction treatment and periods of sobriety should be elucidated. In the case of alcohol or benzodiazepine abuse, withdrawal symptoms should be specifically enquired about.

In an emergency situation, with an acutely ill patient – for example an acutely manic patient – it may be impossible to laboriously tease out previous psychiatric history and this should be left for a later stage once the patient's mood has settled, or obtained from collateral sources. Mood can influence the type of detail that is recalled – for example, a patient with moderate to severe depression may have marked feelings of guilt and may portray themselves in a negative light in terms of past history.

Pearls and Pitfalls

- Lack of insight may impair the patient's ability to provide a detailed account of previous episodes.
- Ask specifically about previous suicide attempts.
- A detailed account of previous treatments will inform the choice of treatment.
- Questioning about substance misuse requires a strategic approach with a high index of suspicion.

Previous Medical History

Obtaining a previous medical history is a logical follow-on from the previous psychiatric history. Many medical illnesses can produce psychiatric symptoms and organic disorder should be ruled out before it is assumed that the illness is entirely functional. Likewise, some psychiatric illnesses and psychotropic medications are associated with medical conditions (for example hypothyroidism and depression, or the association of some antipsychotics with impaired glucose tolerance). The same model should be followed as in a general medical setting. The doctor should enquire about any major medical illnesses or surgeries, and should specifically ask about cardiac problems, hypertension, diabetes, epilepsy and so on. It is remarkable how many patients do not consider hypertension to be a medical illness. Often, patients will comment that they have always been healthy, and have had no reason to visit their doctor, but later reveal that they are taking anti-hypertensives and a statin. When questioned, they will admit to a history of hypertension and hypercholesterolaemia but seem to have little appreciation of the relevance of this. In cases where a patient has developed psychiatric symptoms following an accident, it is important to ask about previous accidents and injuries sustained.

Previous Forensic History

In some cases, it will be important to get a detailed history of any brushes with the law; in other cases it should be obvious that such questioning is not necessary. Those who have had frequent legal entanglements are usually adept at avoiding detailed questioning and minimising their own responsibility for such entanglements. However, it is essential to clearly elucidate the details of any crime committed, and sentences served, as well as periods in remand. Alcohol and drug-related offences should be specifically asked about, particularly where there is a possibility of a substance misuse problem.

Current Medications

The patient should be asked about what medications he is currently taking. It may be helpful to ask him to produce these if they are at hand, as patients often have an inaccurate knowledge of what they are taking. Doctors should have some idea of the colours of commonly prescribed psychotropic medications (for example, the lilac colour of a common formulation of sodium valproate) which may well be of assistance in establishing the patient's medication. A fair amount of detective work may be required for this purpose, often requiring the assistance of a British National Formulary. It may be necessary to run through a range of the trade names of commonly prescribed psychotropic medications in order to jog the patient's memory. Some patients will know their medications by the writing on the tablets – for example, "Roche 5s" (diazepam 5mg) or "D10s" (diazepam 10mgs). Many older patients know lithium as "salt tablets" (as this mood stabiliser was often called lithium salts), although this terminology may also be used to refer to diuretics.

Many patients on psychotropic medications have poor compliance and it is worth checking this when asking in general about medications. Similar principles apply to those used to elucidate alcohol use – the doctor should indicate, through his manner of questioning, that it is not at all unusual, and is quite acceptable, to take one's medication on a sporadic basis only (later of course, emphasising the importance of compliance when it comes to discussing treatment). Patients generally feel guilty about non- and partial compliance and expect a scolding from the doctor.

Family History

The purposes of elucidating family history are to establish the structure of the patient's family of origin to identify any psychiatric disorders suffered by other family members (particularly psychiatric disorders known to be heritable). It may be useful to document a complex family history in graph form. The family history will provide some idea of the patient's early childhood environment as well as his current relationships with his family of origin, and these issues can be explored further under the headings indicated in the next section.

The doctor should first ask the patient about parents and siblings, their state of health or otherwise, and occupation. As always, open questions should be used to avoid false negative answers about others suffering from psychiatric disorders. When asking about an extended family history of psychiatric disorder, the following questioning style has been found useful by this author:

Doctor: Is there anyone in your family who has suffered from any psychological or emotional problems?

Patient: No, I can't think of anyone.

Doctor: What about others outside your immediate family, cousins, aunts, uncles, grandparents?

Patient: Oh, I think my great-aunt died in a mental hospital. But that happened in those days, didn't it? People got put into mental hospitals and didn't come out. I think she had a breakdown after having a baby. There might have been land involved, I don't know.

Doctor: Do you know anything about what she was diagnosed with?

Patient: No, not much.

Doctor: Do you know if she got sick very soon after having her baby, or some weeks later?

Patient: Sorry, I don't know much about it. I suppose you'd have to get the old records from the hospital.

Older patients in particular will be familiar with family members who "suffered from their nerves", a euphemism for mental disorder. It may be useful to ask if anyone was known as the "black sheep" of the family – this may indicate a personality disorder. The majority of the lay public significantly underestimate the prevalence of alcohol dependency syndrome; therefore, obtaining an accurate family history of alcohol problems can be challenging. Rather than asking directly if there are any alcoholics in the family (to most people an alcoholic is a homeless person who drinks from a paper bag), it is generally more fruitful to ask if there is anyone in the family who the patient considers drinks too much, or with whom alcohol does not "agree". More precise, closed questions can then follow once a promising line of questioning suggests itself.

Personal History

The importance of the personal history cannot be underestimated, but often is, particularly by students and trainee psychiatrists. Its purposes are multiple: to establish the patient's early childhood environment and formative relationships with care-givers, the patient's developmental history and academic progress, relationships with peers and ability to form relationships, work history and current social network, as well as religious beliefs, regular activities and interests. This allows the interviewer to establish the patient's formative early environment, to estimate the patient's intelligence, and gain a sense of the patient's personality. While some patients are nonplussed by detailed questioning about their life, for many patients it indicates that the doctor is genuinely interested in them and therefore can form the basis for a therapeutic alliance.

The doctor should commence by asking about what the patient knows of his birth – there is some evidence that obstetric complications are associated with schizophrenia, for example. The patient should then be asked about his early relationships with family members, particularly parents. It takes many years to develop a skilled manner of questioning about these matters, but the novice can nonetheless gain useful information by using open questions and allowing the patient to talk freely. The possible direction such questions might take may have already been suggested by the family history. The following interview illustrates the topics that may arise:

Doctor: "What sort of family home did you grow up in, as a child? You told me already that your father had an alcohol problem."

Patient: "Not a very happy home really...."

Doctor: "Oh? How was that?"

Patient: "Well, because my father drank a lot, my parents fought a lot. My Dad was fine when he wasn't drinking, but he was abusive physically to my Mum and me, because I was the oldest girl. In the end, my Mum got out."

Doctor: "Tell me a little about his abusiveness. How would that show itself?"

Patient: "Well, when he'd come home from the pub he'd be shouting and roaring. He'd go mad if his dinner wasn't on the table. But we never knew what time he'd be home. My Mum would be on tenterhooks. I think it did affect me. But he wasn't an alcoholic, he just drank a lot. Then some Sundays, if he wasn't drinking he'd be in good form and we'd go out. I remember going to the beach and getting ice-cream. But you never knew how he'd be."

Doctor: "That sounds as though it was very difficult at times. What do you think it did to you as a little girl?"

A wide range of issues arise here – the patient's difficult early childhood needs to be explored further, particularly whether or not she identified with her mother, took on the role of care-taker, whether her experiences had a traumatic effect and so on. The depth to which such issues are explored will depend on the context of the interview, the patient's willingness and level of insight, and a range of other factors. In many cases, the effects of childhood adversity will be "unpacked" over several interviews as the therapeutic relationship develops. It may not be appropriate to explore painful topics in depth in an initial interview, although the doctor should not shy away from discussion of such topics where they arise. Many patients will be reluctant to discuss painful childhood memories in an early interview and may deny that their childhood was anything but blissful (this author has heard of more happy childhoods in the context of psychiatric interviews than one would have believed possible).

The topic of sexual abuse is a particularly sensitive one to broach for the inexperienced interviewer. Simply raising the issue of traumatic memories of childhood in the context of the interview may allow the patient to return to the topic at a later stage. My own practice is to ask if anything particularly traumatic happened to the patient as a child. While this question is often met with a denial at first, many patients refer to it later – this question is not forgotten if it is relevant – and will admit to a history of some form of abuse once they have established greater trust in their psychiatrist, over a period of time. Simply raising the question is unlikely to suggest to the patient that something occurred which did not in reality (false memories of this sort usually arise in the context of psychotherapy with a therapist who is overly focussed on sexual abuse). Where there is a history of childhood abuse, simply knowing that the doctor is interested in hearing about it, can open up the possibility of discussing it when the patient feels ready. Of course, emotional and physical abuse may occur without sexual abuse.

Once the patient's relationships with parents has been explored, the interviewer should ask about relationships with other important adults, as well as siblings, and should then ask about the patient's current relationships within their family of origin. This will give the interviewer an idea of the patient's personality as well as his social supports.

It is important to establish whether or not the patient had any birth injury or labour complications – for instance, the latter may be associated with a higher risk of schizophrenia. The patient's developmental milestones should be established – at what age did they walk, talk and so on. Of course, the interviewer needs to know the normal milestones.

It is the convention to ask about so-called childhood neurotic traits such as nail-biting and eneuresis but the value of these in terms of either personality diagnosis or the diagnosis of mental illness is dubious. Of greater importance is the patient's educational history, including their historical relationship with peers and with those in authority. The interviewer should ask what level of education was achieved, including examinations sat and the grades achieved therein, if possible. This may be highly relevant, for instance, where a major mental illness has developed in the teenage years; schizophrenia, for example, may influence cognitive and overall functioning to the degree that the patient's Leaving Certificate results do not match the expectations generated by Junior Certificate results. Likewise, third level education and the performance achieved therein should be explored. Some patients who have not achieved a high level of education – for example, those with primary education only – may be somewhat embarrassed by this, particularly in the presence of a doctor who, in their eyes, has achieved a stellar level of educational achievement. I find it improves the therapeutic relationship to offer the patient a reasonable "excuse" for an early exit from education. For example, many patients who grew up in large families in the 1930s, 40s and 50s or even later, may have had little option but to leave school after primary level in order to earn money for the family. It is important to acknowledge this as a valid reason for leaving education. It may surprise medical students that many pupils dislike school, particularly those who do not excel either academically or in sports. The following form of words avoids embarrassment:

Doctor: "So, how far did you go in your schooling?"
Patient: "Oh, you know, I hated school, I left in third year."
Doctor: "Did you do your Junior Cert or did you decide to go before that?"
(suggesting that this might be perfectly reasonable).
Patient: "Well, I left before my Junior Cert."
Doctor: "Oh, so you went working then, did you?"

Again, the suggestion here is that leaving school early was respectable because the patient was working and earning.

By the same token, it should be easy to spot the patient who has reached a high level of education and questioning may indicate the doctor's assumption that the patient went to third level. This will flatter the articulate patient. These may seem like obvious niceties, but they can make a significant difference in developing a therapeutic relationship with the patient. Those with highly developed Western-style social skills will have an instinctive grasp of these subtle points. Obviously, social mores and conventions will be different in Eastern and other societies, and a truly skilled clinician will need to be able to relate to patients from a wide range of cultures and backgrounds.

The patient should be asked about their ability to form friendships at school, as well as their relationships with teachers and other authority figures. Difficulties in these areas may presage (although not always) later difficulties in sustaining personal relationships or relationships with authority figures in adulthood. It is important to ask if the patient was ever suspended or expelled from school – those who were frequently suspended may well gloss over the fact or minimise their own part in their expulsion. Difficulties at school may indicate a specific learning disability. Some patients give a history suggestive of attention-deficit hyperactivity disorder – including difficulties in concentrating, poor relationships with authority figures – but it is impossible to ascertain this without a clear collateral history, preferably from a teacher. It is surprisingly worthwhile contacting the school of young adult patients – teachers almost always recall past pupils within several years, and may well have identified pupils at risk of developing difficulties in adult life while they were still schoolchildren.

Likewise, third level education should be explored; many patients complete secondary education with relative ease but fall at the hurdle of undergraduate education where there is more self-directed learning and less structure.

A discussion of employment history follows on logically from the educational history. Although it may be tedious, when time allows, employment history is worth exploring in detail. Some patients with personality problems may give a superficially good work history, but become past masters at glossing over interpersonal difficulties at work. They may avoid direct questions about frequent changes of job. It is up to the interviewer to judge whether or not frequent job changes are the norm for the patient's cultural background and training. For instance, it would not be unusual for a junior doctor to change jobs every six months but a similar pattern would be unusual for a secretary. Discovering the real reasons for frequent job changes may take several interviews and the establishment of a good therapeutic relationship. Psychiatric illness may interfere significantly with the person's occupational functioning; it is also important to establish the patient's current level of occupational functioning in the context of current psychopathology.

The patient's interpersonal relationships should be explored in detail. This will give an idea both of the patient's current social supports as well as of their personality. Generally, the focus of most questioning in this regard will be on the patient's relationship with a spouse, parent or child. It is well worth discussing the patient's sexual relationships over the years, although in an acute presentation, it will be less relevant. Again, further detail will generally transpire over the course of treatment and the doctor should avoid accepting everything the patient says at face value. This following example, adapted from real-life clinical practice, illustrates this point:

Doctor (to depressed female patient): *"So, your son John is at home with you and your husband – how do you get on with John?"*

Patient: "Ah, he's grand, a grand fella."

Doctor: "Does he give you a hand with the housework?"

Patient: "Ah, he'll cook a dinner sometimes. He's no bother, just stays in his room mostly."

Doctor: "And is he concerned about your depression?"

Patient: "Oh he is, doctor. He asked me to tell you to give me some of the D10s (diazepam) and some of the DF118s (codeine). For my depression. He said they were very good for it. He didn't think the last diazepams you gave me were strong enough."

It will not surprise the reader to discover that John had a significant substance misuse problem and was regularly in custody for drug-related offences. Patients may be reluctant to paint family members in a negative light and indeed may idealise them.

The patient's relationship with a primary carer should be discussed in detail, as this relationship may well have a significant effect on their prognosis.

Medical undergraduates tend to feel uncomfortable discussing sexual orientation with patients. It should certainly not be assumed that all patients are heterosexual. When a patient is homosexual, it may be obvious from elements in the history and patients will often offer the information readily. Issues regarding sexuality may well be a significant factor in the patient's presenting complaint, for example. Sometimes it is not obvious, even towards the end of the interview, whether a patient is heterosexual or homosexual. The most diplomatic approach is to ask generally about partners, or "any particularly significant relationships"; this approach at least does not cause offence and provides an invitation to the patient to discuss sexual relationships if they wish to. Where a patient is uncertain or conflicted regarding sexual orientation, or indeed gender identity, it is not reasonable to expect that they would discuss these issues without developing trust in the doctor. The doctor should at least indicate by his demeanour that he will not allow his own sexual orientation or moral views impinge on any discussion of the patient's concerns. It should be noted that concerns about sexual orientation arising in late teens or subsequently may be indicative of an underlying psychotic illness (although of course this is not always the case).

Pearls and Pitfalls

- Novice interviewers commonly obtain insufficient information about personal history.
- Several interviews may be required to establish adequate detail about personal history.
- The topic of childhood trauma may be introduced at the initial interview and followed up when trust has been established.
- Doctors have a vicarious and statutory responsibility towards children who may be at risk from a patient.

Where there are young or even teenage children, the doctor has a vicarious duty of care towards the children of his patients (and towards any children who may be in contact with his patients), even if he never actually meets those children. In Ireland and the UK, this is a statutory responsibility under the Childcare Act. Although mental illness is not necessarily associated with child neglect or abuse, it may be – particularly when there is addiction present in a parent – and a referral to a social worker may be warranted. It is important to recognise that for many women, small children are almost an extension of themselves and may be implicated in suicidal ideation. The doctor should therefore be particularly alert to the potential risk to children with a depressed parent. In all cases, the patient's relationships with their children should be discussed.

Additionally, the patient's religious beliefs should be discussed as should their general interests and activities. Asking the patient how they spend their day may yield surprising answers. Some patients with severe and enduring mental illness may have almost no social contact or meaningful activity from day to day but may not readily proffer this information.

Premorbid Personality

It is traditional in a psychiatric interview to ask the patient about their premorbid personality. It is unreasonable to expect that anyone can give an entirely dispassionate view of themselves. This view will at least be coloured by mood – a depressed patient may provide an inaccurately negative view of himself, while a manic patient may give an overinflated and grandiose version of the reality.

In truth, a picture of premorbid personality can be built up from the personal history, from collateral history and from the rapport formed by the patient at interview. The patient's own account of their premorbid personality is but a small part of the information which contributes to this picture.

Mental State Examination

The mental state examination involves observation of the "external" manifestations of the patient's psychopathology. It is not possible to directly observe the patient's thinking processes, for example – but it may be possible to make deductions about that thinking process through the patient's discourse. Essentially, mental state examination involves the observer trying to reach a sense of the patient's subjective state and phenomenology, from one remove. Empathy should not be underestimated in this context. For instance, empathic skills may allow the psychiatrist to gain a subjective sense of the fear that is experienced by a paranoid patient and may therefore put him in a better position to imagine the possible risks associated with this fear.

Much of the mental state examination is, in reality, carried out simultaneously with history-taking. Psychopathology will be the focus of much of the presenting complaint. Only the most unobservant interviewer would fail to notice, after a lengthy interview, the demeanour of a patient who is depressed. The mental state examination serves to deconstruct the various aspects of behaviour, speech and so on that will form the interviewer's general impression. As with history-taking, the mental state examination should be addressed under various headings so that essential information is not missed.

Undergraduates often expect patients with psychiatric illness to be strange or unusual and therefore may fail to observe odd behaviour or an abnormal affect. It may be helpful for the student to imagine how it would feel to talk to the patient at, for instance, a party – this often helps to throw the abnormal aspects of the patient's demeanour into relief, and to make them more visible.

When describing the mental state, a check-list approach should be avoided; a truly meaningful psychiatric formulation should involve not just the presence or absence of – for instance – hallucinations, but a commentary on the patient's way of relating and general personality style. A good mental state examination should therefore make the patient recognisable by the listener when they meet the patient. In this respect, the student or trainee should arm themselves with an extensive vocabulary – the comment that the patient forms a detached rapport with poor eye contact, and little spontaneous speech brings to mind a vivid image of the patient and is far more descriptive than simply commenting that the patient had no psychotic symptoms.

Although a detailed discussion of all types of psychopathology is beyond the scope of this chapter, the following indicates the headings that should be used. The behaviours and other observable phenomena mentioned under each heading are not an exhaustive list. The novice may find it useful to jot these headings down before the interview, in order not to forget vital aspects such as suicidal ideation. None of the behaviours and so on that are discussed are diagnostic in themselves, but taken together in conjunction with historical aspects will support a diagnosis.

It cannot be emphasised enough that the mental state examination applies only to mental phenomena that are present at the time of interview. Phenomena that were present previously, but not now, should be included in the history but not under the heading of mental state.

Appearance and Behaviour

The patient's general appearance should be noted. Patients who are depressed or demented may display poor hygiene and self-care. Clothes buttoned up incorrectly may indicate a dyspraxia. Manic patients may be dressed in inappropriately bright or skimpy clothing. Extensive tattoos may be associated with criminal behaviour and should be noted. In some patients, the level of grooming may be a good reflection of their mood – however, many depressed patients will present as perfectly well-groomed. Occasionally, there may be a bizarre aspect to the patient's appearance that is associated with underlying psychotic symptoms – for example, a patient who presented wrapped in insulation tape in order to prevent his neighbour from sending X-rays into his brain.

Behaviour during the interview may be cooperative and appropriate. The paranoid patient may present as suspicious and unforthcoming; the agitated patient will be restless and unable to settle during the interview. Severely depressed patients may stare at the floor, making little eye contact and sighing throughout the interview. Patients with an elated mood may be disinhibited and intrusive during the interview.

Rapport

Rapport means the quality of the relationship that the patient forms with the interviewer. This will depend on personality, mood, psychotic symptoms and many other factors. Obviously the interviewer should attempt to establish a good rapport with the patient. Anxiety may prevent the patient from easily forming a good rapport initially but this should improve as the interview progresses. Manic patients may initially form an overfamiliar rapport but may become hostile and angry when thwarted. A patient who is guarded and suspicious may be paranoid. Sometimes depressed patients will be too apathetic and unmotivated to form a good rapport.

Speech

The physical qualities of the patient's speech should be noted – rate, volume, pitch, rhythm, and so on. A depressed patient may have monosyllabic, low-pitched, monotonous speech; a manic patient may have pressure of speech with a rapid rate.

Mood

The term mood is generally used to indicate the patient's prevailing subjective "form". This will have been gleaned to a large extent from the history, but the patient's current mood state should be clarified.

Affect

Affect generally indicates the objective manifestations of mood. The two will not necessarily match – for instance, manic patients may complain of a subjectively low mood (often they are in reality describing irritability) while being objectively elated. Sometimes schizophrenia may be associated with an incongruent affect, where the objective manifestations of mood do not match the subjective description, or may be inappropriate for the topic under discussion.

Thought Content

The content of the patient's thoughts will be deduced from the concerns and preoccupations he has already discussed under the heading of presenting complaint. The interviewer must establish whether his concerns are, in fact, delusions (firm fixed false beliefs), ruminations, worries, negative thoughts and so on. The interviewer clearly must be aware of the definitions and characteristics of delusions and other symptoms. Paranoid patients in particular may be guarded and reluctant to discuss their delusions. Many patients, despite lacking insight, will know at some level that if they discuss delusional beliefs, the doctor will not believe them and will deem them unwell. It may therefore be difficult to elicit such ideas directly and the doctor must use skill and subterfuge to elicit them. In practice, this will mean that the doctor has a high index of suspicion from early in the interview and must not miss opportunities offered to explore potential psychotic symptomatology.

Sometimes "fishing" questions may help to reveal delusional beliefs – for example, asking about whether or not the patient has special powers or a special mission, or whether it is possible that someone if attempting to control them in any way. Experienced psychiatrists tend to be more successful in getting "results" from this type of question, which should not be posed in too obvious a manner. Guarded and paranoid patients will be alert to any obvious attempts at discussing core beliefs.

The interviewer must ask specifically about any passivity delusions – this is particularly important when there are good grounds to suspect an underlying psychosis. Care must be taken to distinguish the normal phenomenon of feeling emotionally influenced by others from the concrete passivity experience of literal control of one's thoughts, actions, will and so on.

Although strictly speaking, suicidal and homicidal ideation are aspects of thought content, they are well worth habitually considering under a separate heading. This guarantees that the interviewer will not forget to ask! Such ideation may have been part of the presenting complaint, and therefore may already have been discussed in detail. Where it has not already been discussed, it may be helpful to introduce the idea of suicidal ideation gradually, starting with questions about general negative thinking, feelings of futility and slowly coming around towards the topic of suicidal ideas and intent. Where such ideation is present, it should be discussed in detail to establish whether or not the patient is at risk to himself. Contrary to popular myth, patients will not be made to attempt suicide by asking such questions: most patients are relieved to discuss the topic. Homicidal ideation is somewhat more difficult to introduce as a topic, but should not be neglected, particularly in the context of psychosis and in moderate to severe depression, where homicidal ideas about loved ones may be an extension of suicidal ideation.

Thought Form

Thought form cannot be assessed directly and is deduced from the flow of speech. Thought form may be significantly distorted in schizophrenia; this is known as formal thought disorder. The novice should attempt to interview patients with formal thought disorder whenever the opportunity arises (such opportunities arise most frequently in inpatient units or other acute settings) as this phenomenon tends to respond rapidly to antipsychotic medication and therefore may be short-lived. The interviewer who meets a patient with thought disorder will find that he is unable to describe the conversation in retrospect, although some aspects of it appeared to make sense at the time. There are various sub-phenomena within the category of formal thought disorder which are described in detail in books on psychopathology. It is well worth writing down examples as they occur in the interview, as they will be forgotten afterwards but will help support a diagnosis.

Patients with elated mood may present with pressure of speech – rapid speech which gives the impression that the patient has multiple ideas which he cannot express quickly enough.

Circumstantiality – "beating around the bush" – can be distinguished from formal thought disorder in that the patient will eventually get to the point after a long-winded discussion, whereas the patient with formal thought disorder will be unable to retain in their mind the ultimate point of the story.

Perceptual Abnormalities

This category includes illusions, pseudohallucinations and hallucinations. Of these, hallucinations have the most diagnostic significance. Sometimes, patients may be obviously responding to hallucinations during the interview. Hallucinations have the vivid, concrete quality of perceptions based on real external stimuli; however, as with delusional beliefs, patients may deny that they are present. The full range of sensory modalities may be experienced in hallucinations and should be asked about. The content of hallucinations should be enquired about– for example, with auditory hallucinations, what the voices say, who is speaking, whether second person or third person and so on.

Insight

The patient's level of insight will generally become evident as the interview progresses. Insight is a dynamic rather than a static phenomenon and may change with treatment of a mental disorder; in some cases, however, it may not change at all. Insight can be considered at a range of different levels. For example, at the basic level, insight may amount simply to the patient recognising that he is unwell. A very sophisticated level of insight would involve the patient being able to formulate his own difficulties in terms of the interaction of psychological factors (even unconscious factors) and social factors as well as illness. This very sophisticated level of insight is uncommon. Many psychotic patients will completely lack insight. Insight is a key aspect of the mental state in addictions and eating disorders – denial may be used as a defence mechanism in these cases, and often mitigates against the patient fully recognising the seriousness of their difficulties. For example, an alcohol dependent patient may assert that he drinks because his wife is so unaffectionate, failing (or refusing) to recognise that her lack of affection may stem from his drinking!

Motivation

As with insight, motivation is a dynamic phenomenon and may change for a range of reasons. In acute psychiatric presentations such as depression, elated mood, psychosis and so on, motivation may not be the most important aspect of mental state, but increases in importance as the patient's illness improves and he develops some ability to assist in his own recovery. Motivation is of particular importance in addictions and eating disorders and will be one of the most important factors in predicting recovery. Generally speaking, the interviewer will develop an impression of the patient's motivation as the interview progresses – direct questioning regarding motivation may yield limited information.

Cognitive Function

The assessment of cognitive function is beyond the scope of this chapter. There are a number of easily administered screening questionnaires which may be useful. Significant cognitive deficits may be obvious from the interview itself. Most screening questionnaires touch on a range of cognitive functions such as registration, recall and attention but more detailed assessment by a neuropsychologist may be required for greater diagnostic precision. The interviewer should attempt to make a general assessment of the patient's intelligence – this can be guessed from the patient's educational and occupational level, use of language, and general perspicacity – although of course none of these factors alone are diagnostic of any specific intelligence level.

Pearls and Pitfalls

- Many aspects of mental state examination may be gleaned in the course of the interview.
- While key headings should be used, a checklist approach should be avoided.
- Risks such as those of suicide and homicide should be actively considered in the context of mental state examination.

Presenting the Case History and Mental State Examination

Just as there is an art to the psychiatric interview, so there is an art to editing and presenting the relevant information in a concise, meaningful way which supports a particular differential diagnosis. The doctor or student will have formed his own differential diagnosis which he should arrange in order of probability. The case history and mental state should support this differential. It is up to the person presenting the case to suggest to the listener – by the material and the way in which it is presented – what differential diagnosis he is considering. A good presenting complaint should include all relevant symptoms, as well as relevant negatives; judicious but not excessive quotation from the patient will bring the case history to life, support the diagnosis, and, most importantly, keep examiners awake.

It is not enough to simply present material as it has arisen in the interview – the interviewer's job is to edit and collate the material under the relevant headings. The following example displays a good grasp of the principles of case presentation:

Mr. X describes a three month history of "feeling upset" with disturbed sleep. While he does not describe a low mood, he has been distressed by hearing the voice of his next-door neighbour talking about him, when he had thought he was alone in the house. He describes his neighbour saying "he's gay". In the last few weeks, he has become aware that his neighbour is in communication with the police to have him arrested. He believes that his neighbour is controlling his thoughts through the gas meter. He told me "he can hear my thoughts when he turns on his own gas heating. He's doing it just so that he can listen to my thoughts. That way he can change them the way he wants."

In the past week he has been housebound as he is terrified to leave his house in case he meets his neighbour.

While the above is only an extract, it indicates clearly that the doctor has considered whether this could be a depressive illness, but thinks that it is more likely to be a primary psychotic illness. The doctor has selected a highly relevant bit of psychopathology, quoting a vivid example of thought broadcasting (and possibly thought insertion) which brings the narrative to life. Extensive and unedited quoting tends to have the opposite effect however – it is soporific to the listener and suggests that the interviewer has not done the intellectual work that it is involved in psychiatric diagnosis, but is leaving it to the examiner or listener.

Information may not necessarily arise during the interview in the order of the headings already suggested above, but should be rearranged in terms of those headings. This will allow the case presentation to flow logically and will build a picture of the patient which is then rounded off, as it were, by the mental state examination. As commented above, a good mental state examination should make the patient immediately recognisable to the examiner when the patient enters the room, and therefore requires far more than a checklist approach to psychopathology.

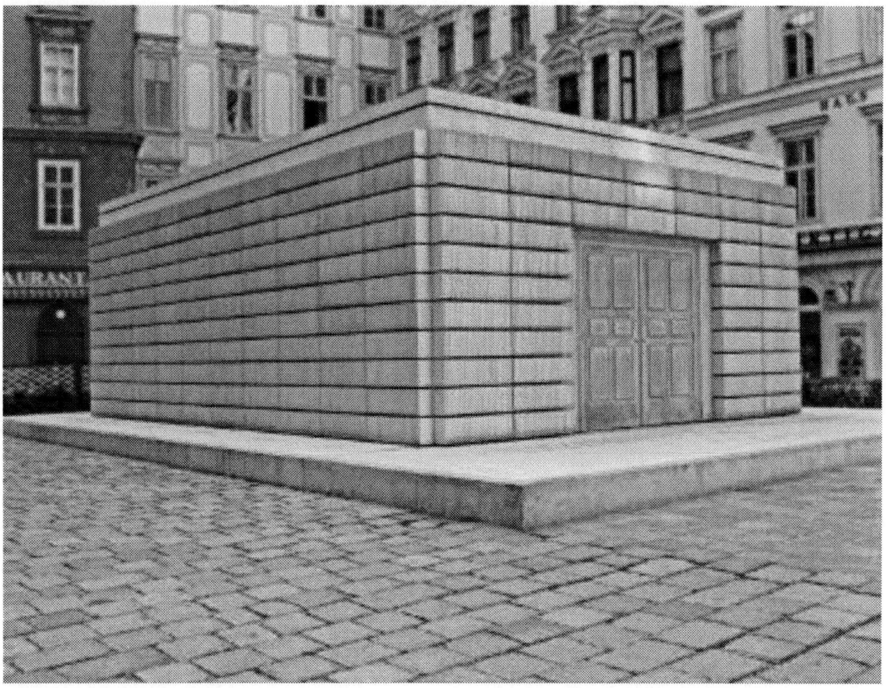

The Judenplatz Holocaust Memorial (The Nameless Library). Rachel Whiteread 2000. Source: eigene Fotografie, August 2005*Photographer: Hans Peter Schaefer, http://www.reserv-a-rt.de.

The case presentation should end with both a differential diagnosis and a formulation. Formulation is beyond the scope of this chapter but involves collating the biological, psychological and social predisposing, precipitating and perpetuating factors in order to develop an understanding of the patient and his illness: although it is a source of considerable anxiety to trainee psychiatrists, it is simply the expression of the thinking process of a competent psychiatrist, and the logical result of an intelligent approach to history-taking.

Rachel Whiteread's Holocaust memorial in the Vienna Judenplatz is simultaneously compact, discreet, unobtrusive, emotive and weighty. The outside of the memorial is shaped not from the spines of books, as one might expect from a library, but from the opposite side, from their pages. This is a reference to the Jews as "People of the Book", but also suggests something hidden. There are no names on the outside – and there are no doors. The memorial sums up the weight of history and trauma and reflects the manner in which history and trauma can be concealed, unlocked only by the most subtle questioning. An apparently plain exterior can conceal a vast array of memories – the moment in which the history is revealed is brief, and must be grasped as it is revealed by the keen and sensitive listener. This is not to imply that all patients with psychiatric disorders have been traumatised, or that taking a psychiatric history involves a forensic uncovering of the patient's past – but to remind the clinician that our patients are inevitably more complex than they initially appear.

In: Learning Clinical Skills
Editors: Bridget Maher and Pat Henn
ISBN: 978-1-62100-409-7

Chapter XX

Ophthalmology for Medical Students

Sinead Byrne

Clinical Case

A 28 year old male attends the Eye Casualty Department complaining of mild ocular discomfort, mild visual blurring and photosensitivity in the right eye. The left eye is entirely asymptomatic. These symptoms have been present for a day and began shortly after the patient returned home from work. The patient had no significant ocular history of note, never wore glasses, was medically fit and well, and was not taking any medications. On further questioning, it was noted that the patient had been hammering a nail into a wooden block at work that day. He was a carpenter by profession. He recalled a large piece of wood flying up and hitting him over the eye but was unaware of any metallic foreign body striking him. Notably, he was not wearing protective eye wear at the time of the injury.

Clinical Examination: The patient's visual acuity was measured using a Snellen chart. It was noted to be 6/9 unaided in the right eye and 6/6 in the left. No improvement was noted in the right eye with pinhole correction. Pupil examination was normal with no evidence of a Relative Afferent Pupil Defect (RAPD). Ophthalmoscopy revealed mild conjunctival injection of the right eye. Both corneae appeared clear with no evidence of corneal perforation. Dilated fundoscopy was normal. There was no evidence of an intra-ocular foreign body on clinical examination.

Student Dilemma

- How can I be sure that this red eye is due to blunt trauma only?
- Is there something more sinister going on?
- Is this type of injury significant?
- What investigations will help me?

Reflection

Not all red eyes are due to conjunctivitis - be suspicious if a red eye is associated with a drop in visual acuity as most 'benign' causes will not cause any visual disturbance. A careful history is essential. Always specifically ask about trauma. The type of trauma is also important as certain injuries are more likely to result in ocular penetration. For example, the velocity of a foreign body resulting from hammering is far greater than that generated by angle-grinding, therefore have a low index of suspicion that an object may have penetrated the eye if the patient gives a history of hammering, especially if no protective eye wear was used. These patients should have ocular imaging (X Ray or CT of orbits) to outrule the presence of a potentially sight threatening intraocular foreign body.

The Ophthalmic Examination –Introduction

A complete ophthalmic examination involves assessing not only the eyeball or globe but also the adjacent anatomical areas in the face, eyebrows, eyelids, lacrimal system, ocular muscles, optic nerve and all the intracranial neurological components of the visual system back to the visual cortex.

Many medical conditions may exhibit their presenting symptoms and signs in the eye and indeed there is often overlap with other medical specialties in caring for ophthalmic patients. It is therefore important that non-ophthalmic practitioners are able to take an accurate ophthalmic history and perform a systematic examination of the eye and visual system.

Ophthalmic History

A careful and accurate history is of great importance as it is likely to suggest a particular part of the eye or visual system that may need particular attention during the ophthalmic examination, and is also likely to dictate some relevant investigations. The ophthalmic history is structured in a similar way to any medical history and begins with a history of the presenting complaint.

History of the Presenting Complaint

Although the spectrum of ocular disease is vast, the number of ophthalmic symptoms that the patient presents with comes from a relatively small list. These include:

- Reduction in visual acuity (may be gradual or, more worryingly, acute).
- Redness of the eye, which may or may not be associated with discharge.
- Double vision (diplopia).
- Pain.

Occasionally, patients are entirely asymptomatic and are referred by another health professional, often an Optometrist, who has detected an abnormality on routine sight testing. A relevant history for each of the common ophthalmic presentations is outlined below (Figures 1- 4).

Whatever the presenting complaint, it is important to determine the nature of its onset, gradual or acute, how long the symptom has been present, and whether it occurs constantly or intermittently. It is also important to ask the patient how the symptom is impacting on their daily life as not all patients with cataract, for example, will be troubled, and therefore surgical intervention is not always indicated.

Common Presenting Complaints in Ophthalmology

Acute Visual Loss

- *Nature of onset* - sudden (usually vascular - often arterial) or transient and recurrent (often embolic)
- *Quantity of visual loss* - profound loss (usually suggests arterial occlusion)
- *Area of vision affected* - central (usually macular) or peripheral (retinal detachment, vascular occlusion or migraine), loss of left or right field (hemianopia)
- *Associated symptoms* - pain, nausea, vomiting, red eye (acute glaucoma), pain on eye movement, peripheral parasthesia (optic neuritis), jaw claudication, headache, weight loss, myalgia (giant cell arteritis), scintillating scotomata and headache (migraine)
- *General medical history* - vascular, rheumatological, neurological, endocrine disease

Gradual Visual Loss

- *Duration of onset* - months to years (cataract, dry ARMD)
- *Worse for distance* (nuclear sclerotic cataract) or near (posterior subcapsular cataract or ARMD)
- *General medical history* - diabetes (cataract or diabetic retinopathy/ maculopathy), multiple sclerosis (optic neuritis)
- *Medications*-steroids (cataract/glaucoma), chloroquine/tamoxifen (maculopathy), chlorpromazine, amiodarone (retinopathy)

Figure 1. Visual Loss.

Unilateral or Bilateral

- *Unilateral* - keratitis, iritis, trauma, sub-conjunctival haemorrhage, acute glaucoma
- *Bilateral* - ocular allergy, bacterial conjunctivitis

Previous Ocular and medical history

- *Contact lens wear* - predisposes to corneal infection (keratitis) and corneal abrasion
- *Previous ocular disease* - many conditions are recurrent (herpetic keratitis, iritis)
- *Medical history* - ankylosing spondylitis, sarcoidosis, inflammatory bowel disease (iritis), seborrheic dermatitis (blepharitis), atopy

Type of Discharge

- *Watery* - viral infection
- *Mucoid* - allergy
- *Purulent* - bacterial infection
- *Copious mucopurulent* - chlamydial, gonoccocal infection

Reduced visual acuity

- *Reduced visual acuity* - acute glaucoma, trauma, iritis
- *Normal visual acuity* - allergic and bacterial conjunctivitis, sub conjunctival haemorrhage

Figure 2. Red Eye.

Constant or intermittent

- Constant diplopia (nerve palsy)
- Intermittent (thyroid eye disease, myasthenia gravis)
- Vascular risk factors (cranial nerve palsy)
- Trauma (fourth nerve palsy)

Monocular or Binocular

- *Binocular diplopia* - two clear images seen when both eyes open, when one eye is occluded only one image is seen (caused by ocular misalignment, cranial nerve palsy)
- *Monocular diplopia* - two images are seen following occlusion of one eye (corneal disease, cataract)

Vertical or Horizontal

- *Horizontal-* if images are beside each other (usually sixth nerve palsy)
- *Vertical* above each other (often third or fourth nerve palsy)

General History

- Thyroid dysfunction
- Muscle fatigability, phonation or breathing difficulty (myasthenia gravis)
- Vascular risk factors (cranial nerve palsy)
- Trauma (fourth nerve palsy)

Figure 3. Diplopia.

Severity of symptoms

- *Mild to moderate irritation* (blepharitis, dry eye, allergy)
- *Pain* (scleritis, keratitis, iritis or raised intraocular pressure)

Associated symptoms

- *Reduced vision* - indicates a more sinister cause (scleritis, acute glaucoma, iritis)
- *Crusting of lids* (blepharitis)
- *Intolerance of dry atmosphere* (dry eye)
- *Discharge* (blepharitis)

Previous Medical and Ocular History

- *Contact lens wear* - dry eye, ocular irritation, corneal abrasion or keratitis (pain)
- *Regular use of eye drops* - allergy and irritation (benzalkonium chloride intolerance)
- *Medical conditions* - thyroid dysfunction (ocular irritation) connective tissue disease (scleritis, keratitis), atopy (ocular irritation)

Figure 4. Irritable/Painful Eyes.

Past Ocular History

It is important to determine whether the patient has a history of any eye disease as many ocular conditions are recurrent, and therefore knowing about previous problems can shed light on the current one. Longstanding use of eye drops can also predispose the patient to certain symptoms such as ocular irritation (benzalkonium chloride sensitivity) or glaucoma as can be the case with long term, unsupervised topical steroid use. A history of any previous eye surgery or trauma should also be sought. Specifically, previous trauma can predispose the patient to the development of cataract, glaucoma or retinal detachment.

A full optical history must also be obtained, asking specifically about wearing of spectacles for distance and near. It is important to determine whether the patient has had an updated refraction (sight test) so as not to confuse reduced visual acuity with uncorrected refractive error. The patient must also be asked about a history of 'lazy eye' or amblyopia since childhood.

Family History

Some ocular conditions have a genetic predisposition - in certain cases a simple pattern of inheritance is demonstrated, while in others, the pattern of inheritance is less well defined. Glaucoma, for example, has a multi-factorial pathogenesis but genetics are known to play a role. Those with a first degree relative with glaucoma are at a significantly higher risk of developing glaucoma themselves and therefore need to be screened on a yearly basis. [1]

Table 1. Ophthalmic History–Relevant Medical Conditions

Vascular History
- Diabetes
- Smoking
- Hypertension
- Ischaemic heart disease (angina pectoris)
- Peripheral vascular disease (intermittent claudication)
- Cholesterol status

Neurological History
- CVA
- Multiple sclerosis
- Myasthenia gravis
- Parkinson's disease

Endocrine History
- Thyroid dysfunction
- Hormonal abnormalities (pituitary dysfunction)

Rheumatological History
- Rheumatoid arthritis
- Wegener's granulomatososis
- Polyarteritis nodosa
- SLE
- Relapsing polychondritis
- Systemic sclerosis
- Polymyalgia rheumatica

General Medical History

Certain medical conditions may have ocular manifestations (diabetes mellitus, thyroid dysfunction, multiple sclerosis) while other medical conditions may need to be specifically considered when treating the ophthalmic patient. For example, before commencing treatment for glaucoma, it is important to take a detailed medical history to ensure that the patient does not suffer from obstructive airways disease or cardiac conduction defects which could be exacerbated by the use of topical beta blockers, commonly used in the treatment of chronic glaucoma. Similarly, when listing a patient for cataract surgery, it is important to ask about any respiratory or arthritic conditions which could preclude the patient from lying flat during their operation. Specific medical conditions which are particularly relevant to the ophthalmic history are listed below (Table 1).

Current Medications

A list of all topically applied eye drops and systemic medications should be obtained. Continued use of topically applied eye drops can result in ocular irritation which is often caused by the preservative, benzalkonium chloride. The use of topical steroid may exacerbate a herpes simplex corneal infection and increase intraocular pressure in predisposed individuals.

A list of all systemic medications must also be documented. Systemic steroids may expedite the onset and progression of cataract, rifabutin and cidofovir may cause uveitis, tamoxifen, chloroquine, chlorpromazine and nitrofurantoin may cause retinal toxicity, and ethambutol, amiodarone and vigabatrin may cause toxic optic neuropathy.

It is also important to document the use of oral anticoagulant medication such as aspirin, warfarin or clopidogrel as this may affect planning of ophthalmic surgical procedures.

Social History

Certain occupations may predispose patients to ocular disease or injury. It is important to obtain a full history regarding the patient's job and lifestyle (smoking, alcohol and diet). Any recent foreign travel must be specifically asked about, as it may yield clues regarding unusual ocular infections or causes of uveitis. An account of the patient's home circumstances must be obtained when listing a patient for a surgical procedure, as day case surgery and post operative care may pose problems for people living alone.

Ophthalmic Examination

A detailed and accurate ophthalmic history can give the practitioner clues as to which part of the ocular system may need particular attention.

Visual Acuity - Snellen Acuity

Visual acuity is a measure of the ability of the eye to see that two closely positioned objects are actually separate. The angle subtended at the normal eye by these two objects is on average 1 minute of arc. Letters on the Snellen chart are constructed as multiples of this angle. This test is performed at 6 metres in Europe and 20 feet in the United States.

A patient who can only see the top letter on the Snellen chart is said to have 6 over 60 vision in that eye. That means that the patient is seeing at six metres what a 'normal' seeing eye would see at 60 metres. The 6/6 line is considered 'normal' visual acuity but in reality, many patients can see the 6/5 or even the 6/4 line which is even better. The number above the line describes the distance the patient is situated from the Snellen chart. The number below the line denotes the lowest line on the chart that the patient can see. On the 6/6 line, each letter is constructed to subtend an angel of 1 minute of arc at a testing distance of 6 metres. On the 6/18 line, each letter subtends an angle of 3 minutes of arc. Each line is constructed in a similar way so that letters on the 6/18 line subtend an angle of 1 minute of arc if tested at 18 metres. Before performing any examination, the examiner must explain clearly to the patient what exactly the examination involves, and obtain the patient's permission before proceeding.

Measuring Snellen Visual Acuity

- Position the patient at 6 metres from the chart.
- If the patient wears distance glasses, these must be worn for the test.
- Occlude the left eye with an occluder and test the right eye.
- Ask the patient to read down as far as possible with the right eye.
- If the vision is less than 6/9, recheck using a pinhole (this compensates for any uncorrected refractive error).
- If the vision is worse than 6/60, the patient is moved 3 metres closer to the chart - if the top line is read the vision is recorded as 3/60.
- If at 3 metres the top letter can not be read, the patient is moved to 1 metre from the chart - if the top letter is now read the vision is recorded as 1/60.
- If at 1 metre the top letter is not seen, the examiner holds up fingers in front of each eye and if the number of fingers is correctly seen, the vision is recorded as 'counting fingers' or CF vision.
- If CF vision cannot be seen, the examiner's hand is moved in front of each eye independently while occluding the other - if the movement is seen the vision is recorded as hand movement or HM vision, noting the distance at which the movement was seen.
- If HM vision is not seen, a bright torch is shone into the eye from various angles and if seen, perception of light or PL vision is recorded and the direction from which the light was shone - superior, inferior, temporal or nasal and the distance from the eye at which the light was shone.
- If the patient is unable to see the light, the vision is recorded as no perception of light or NPL vision.

- If a patient is illiterate, the illiterate E test may be used - the patient is asked to indicate with his finger in which direction the E is facing.

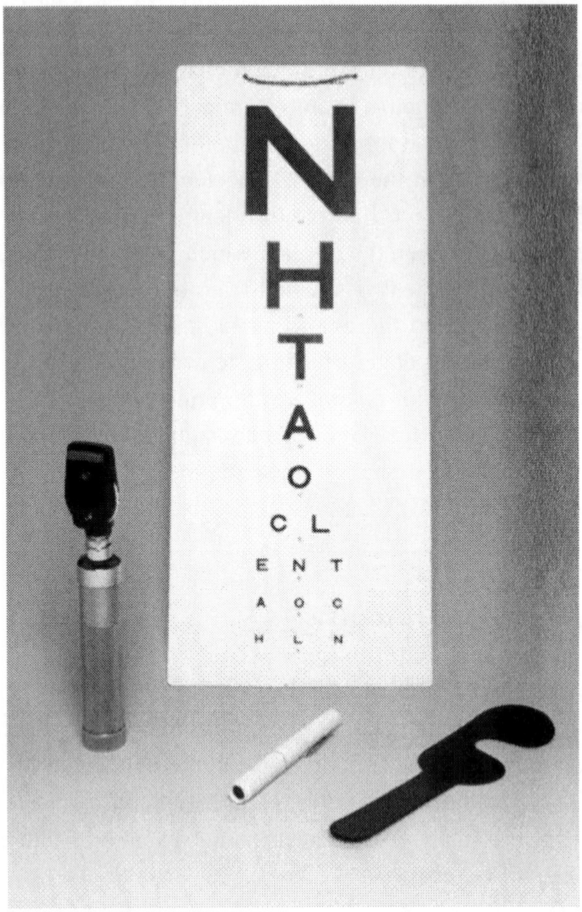

Figure 5. Snellen Visual Acuity Chart.

LogMar Vision

This test is increasingly used for checking children's vision and examining patients with poor visual acuity and contrast sensitivity. The test is performed with the patient situated four metres from the chart.

The LogMar chart has 10 lines with each line containing 5 letters. Each letter has an equal value of 0.02 Logmar units. If the patient can read 3 out of 5 letters on the line, the score for that line is taken and 0.02 LogMar is added for each letter that is not seen. The higher the score, the worse the vision. A LogMar score of 0 is normal vision and equivalent to 6/6 on the Snellen chart. A LogMar score of 1.0 is equal to 6/60 Snellen equivalent.

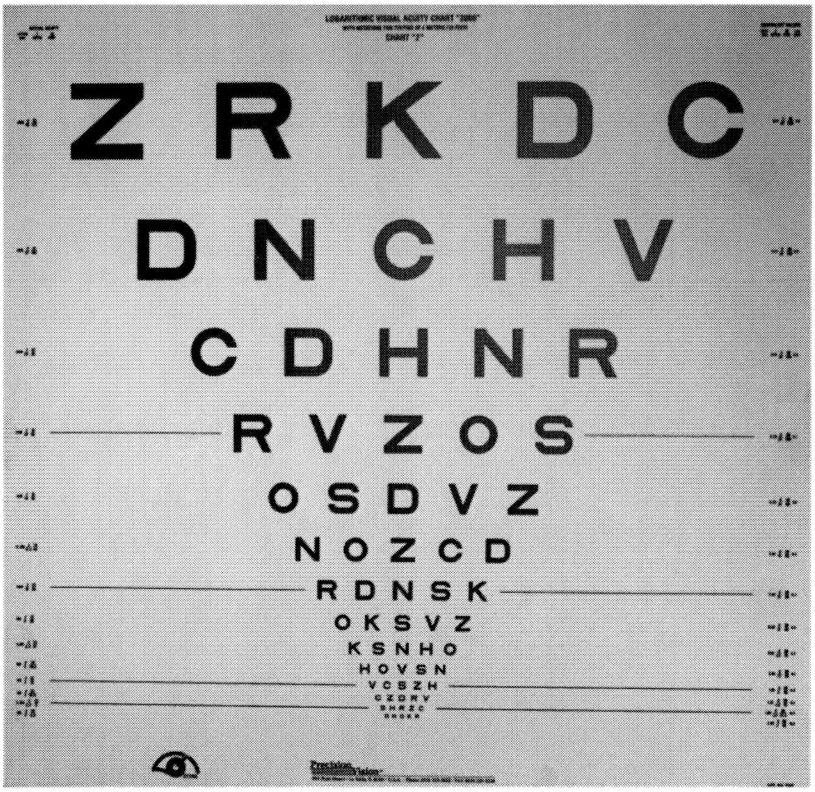

Figure 6. Logmar Visual Acuity Chart.

Near Vision Testing

This should be performed using normal reading correction, if appropriate, and ensuring that adequate ambient lighting is provided.

- Each eye is tested separately.
- The patient holds the near test chart at a comfortable reading distance, usually one third of a metre.
- The smallest print that can be read is recorded - with N5 being the smallest and N48 being the largest.
- N8 is the most common size print in books.

Ophthalmic Examination Techniques

A complete basic ocular examination involves a systematic evaluation of the visual fields to confrontation, pupil responses, cover testing and extra-ocular movement examination and examination of the anterior and posterior segments of the eye.

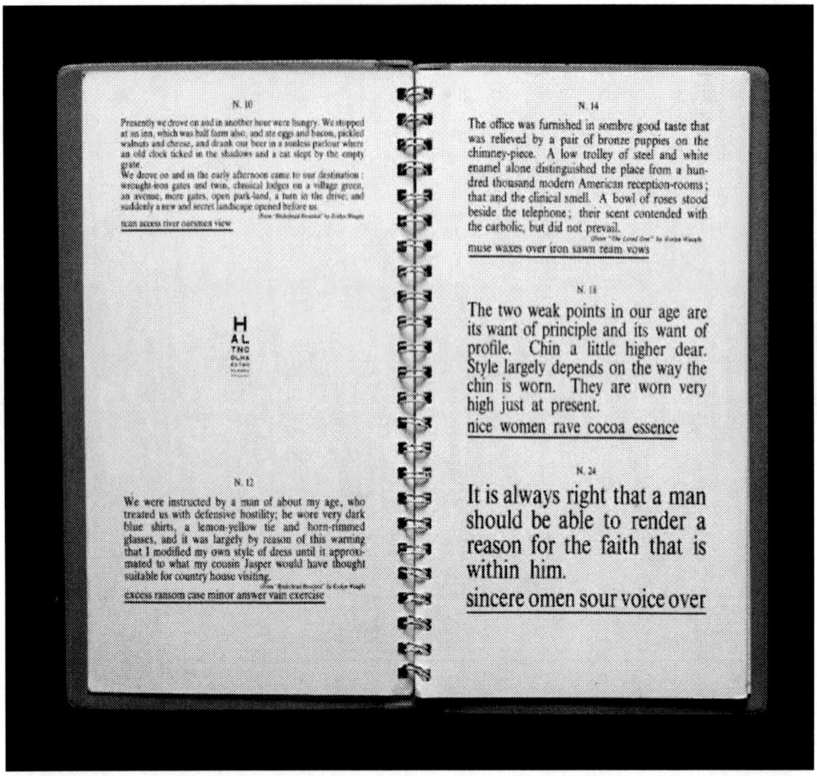

Figure 7. Near Vision Test Chart.

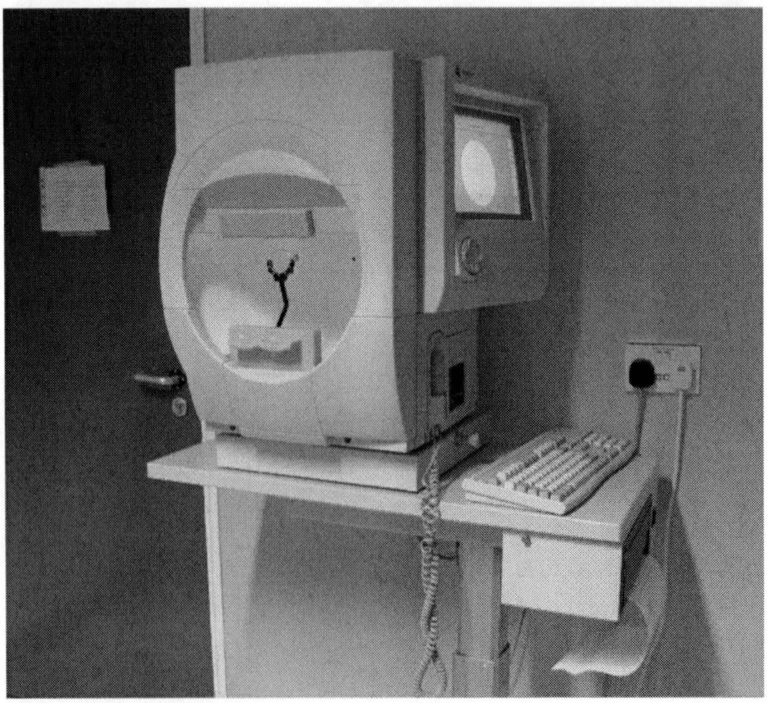

Figure 8. Humphrey Visual Field Analyser.

Visual Field Testing

The visual field is a map representing the patient's visual pathway from the retina to the visual cortex. Different patterns of field loss are seen with abnormalities in different parts of the visual pathway. There is a blind spot temporally in each field which represents the point of exit of the optic nerve from the eye. Confrontational fields are useful at detecting large defects such as hemianopic field defects. Automated perimetry performed in the eye clinic may be needed to detect more subtle defects. The procedure for examining the visual field using confrontational testing, where the patient's field is compared to that of the examiner's presumably normal field, is outlined below.

Confrontational Visual Field Testing

- A red hat pin is ideally used to perform the test.
- Show this to the patient before commencing the test so that the patient knows what to look for.
- If the hat pin can not be seen, then a pen torch or the examiner's finger may be used as alternatives.
- The test is performed at a distance of 1 metre.
- The examiner's eyes and the patient's eyes must be at the same level.
- The right eye is examined first by asking the patient to completely occlude the left eye with his hand.
- Ask the patient if they can see all of your face and shoulders or if any bits are missing or blurred - this helps to detect large hemianopic defects.
- Then ask the patient to fixate on your nose and to say when the moving target first comes into their peripheral field of view.
- Bring the target in from the supero-temporal, supero-nasal, infero-nasal and infero-temporal directions.
- The test is a comparison between the examiner's (presumably normal) field and the patient's - so assuming that both fields are normal, the moving target should be seen by both parties at the same time.

Pupil Examination

Pupil abnormalities are an indicator of extensive retinal disease, optic nerve or chiasmal pathology. To fully understand pupil abnormalities, it is important to be familiar with the anatomy of the neural pathway involved in both the light response and accommodation, a detailed description of which may be found elsewhere. [2]

A bright light is necessary for pupil assessment and the procedure of pupil examination is outlined below.

General Principles of Pupil Examination

- Inspect the pupils for any abnormality in shape or difference in size (anisocoria).
- If the pupil size differs between the two eyes, the pupils should be checked in both dim and bright conditions to determine which is the abnormal pupil.
- If the difference is greater in dim light, then the smaller pupil is abnormal (Horner's syndrome, pharmacological, posterior synechiae).
- If the difference is greater in bright light, then the larger pupil is abnormal (third nerve palsy, Adie's pupil, trauma, pharmacological).
- If the difference is the same in both ambient lighting conditions, the patient has physiological anisocoria.
- Check the direct response, the consensual response and for a relative afferent pupil defect.

The Direct and Consensual Light Response

- This is the response of the pupil being tested to bright light.
- The examiner sits opposite the patient at arm's length.
- Ask the patient to stare at a point in the distance to avoid accommodation.
- The light is shone into the patient's right eye and pupillary constriction is observed - this is referred to as the direct light pupil response.
- While shining the light into the right eye, observe constriction of the left pupil - this is referred to as the consensual light response.
- The consensual light response occurs due to decussation of pupil fibres at the optic chiasm.

Swinging Flashing Light Test

- This detects the presence of a relative afferent pupil defect (RAPD).
- A RAPD indicates the presence of unilateral optic nerve pathology or less commonly, extensive retinal disease.
- A bright light source must be used as abnormalities can be subtle.
- Shine a light in the right eye and watch for the direct response (see above).
- Quickly switch the light to the left eye - the left pupil now constricts due to the direct response but under normal circumstances the right pupil should remain constricted due to the consensual response.
- If one pupil dilates as the light is been swung from one to the other, this denotes a problem with either the retina or the optic nerve on that side.

Testing the Near Response – Accommodation

- This is only necessary if the light response is abnormal.
- The examiner asks the patient to look from distance fixation to a small accommodative target brought towards the patient's eye slowly.
- Both pupils should constrict equally.
- If the response to near is better than to light, this is called light-near dissociation (Adie's tonic pupil, Argyl-Robertson pupil, dorsal midbrain syndrome, amyloidosis, diabetes).

Ocular Motility Examination

This involves assessing both the position of the eyes (cover testing) and the eye movements, which consist of both smooth pursuit movements and saccades. Particular attention should be paid to this part of the examination in children presenting with a squint or patients complaining of double vision.

A. The Cover-Uncover Test

This test is used to detect a manifest squint.

- The examiner should observe to see if one eye is preferred for fixation.
- The patient is asked to look at a fixation target.
- Occlude the eye that is fixing and watch for movement of the other eye - inward movement denotes a divergent strabismus while outward movement denotes presence of a convergent strabismus.
- Now remove the occluder and watch for movement of the eye previously under cover.
- The test is performed for distance and near as certain abnormalities are more clearly demonstrated at different testing distances.

B. The Alternate Cover Test

This test is used to detect a latent squint. If the patient has straight eyes on cover testing, a latent squint may still be present.

- The patient is asked to fixate on an object.
- Cover one eye with an occluder.
- Move the occluder to the other eye.
- Observe the movement of the occluded eye as the cover is taken away.
- Subtle inward movements of the eyes denotes an exophoria and outward movement of the eyes denotes an esophoria.
- A latent squint may become manifest during examination.

C. Eye Movement Examination

Both smooth pursuit and saccadic eye movements should be tested. The procedure is outlined below.

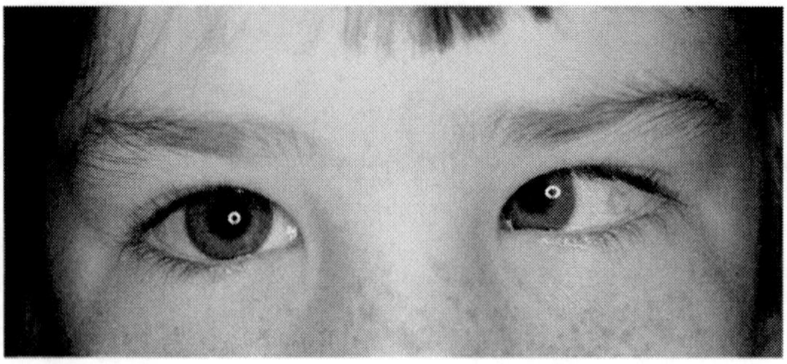

Figure 9. Patient with a left convergent squint.

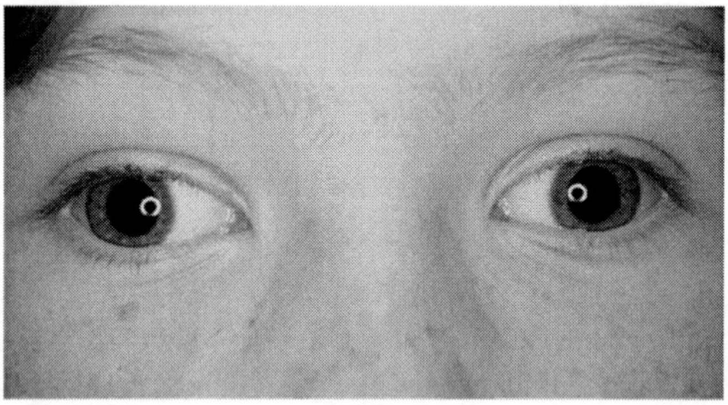

Figure 10. Patient with a right divergent squint.

Examining Smooth Pursuit Eye Movements

- The patient is first observed for any obvious abnormal head posture which can give clues to underlying pathology.
- The examiner then observes for any evidence of nystagmus or 'wobbly eyes'.
- Smooth pursuit movements are checked using a pen torch.
- The examiner sits at arm's length from the patient.
- Ask the patient to look at the light and ask whether one or two lights are seen.
- If two lights are perceived, the examiner asks whether these are beside each other (horizontal diplopia) or above or below each other (vertical/torsional) diplopia.
- If two lights are seen, one eye is then occluded - if now only one image is seen, true binocular diplopia is demonstrated. If two images persist, monocular diplopia is diagnosed.
- The patient is then asked to follow the light into the nine cardinal positions of gaze.

Examining Saccadic Eye Movements

- This test checks for any inter or supra-nuclear eye movement abnormality.
- This test is performed using the examiner's finger and a pen.
- The examiner sits at arm's length from the patient.
- The pen is held in the examiner's right hand and the examiner holds up his left index finger.
- The patient is asked to look quickly between the pen and the finger in both the horizontal and vertical directions.
- This test is useful at detecting gaze palsies and internuclear ophthalmoplegia.

Examination of the Outer Eye: The Ocular Adnexae and Anterior Segment

The Ocular Adnexae: It is important to approach this part of the examination in a systematic way and while the anatomical area to be examined is relatively small, it is important not to overlook any individual component.

Either a pen torch or a direct ophthalmoscope provides adequate illumination. It is important to allow extra time for examination of children or elderly patients, and to always explain carefully what the examination will involve. The examiner should wash his hands thoroughly before commencing this part of the examination.

The examination begins with inspection of the face, especially the periocular area. Any abnormality is documented or, ideally, photographed. A general overview of the patient's appearance, including age, race, nutritional status and mobility can yield useful clues to underlying ocular problems. A checklist of observations is listed below.

Checklist of Observations

The Face

- *Acne rosacea* -blepharitis, dry eye
- *Seborrhoeac dermatitis* -meibomian gland dysfunction, dry eye
- *Bruising* - signs of trauma
- *Rash* - atopy - allergic eye disease, cataract
- *Port-wine discolouration* -Sturge-Weber, glaucoma
- *Unusual facies* (beaking of the nose (scleroderma), flat nasal bridge (Stickler syndrome)

The Eyelids

- Position - Ectropion (out turning of the lid), entropion (in turning of lid) or ptosis (drooping of lid).
- Loss of lashes (cutaneous malignancy).

- Swelling.
- Lumps or bumps
- Rash

The Anterior Segment

This refers to that part of the eye that lies anterior to the iris. It may be examined using a pen torch or ideally a direct ophthalmoscope. Within an eye clinic setting, a slit lamp or binocular microscope is used, although this instrument is often not available to the non ophthalmic practitioner.

Most direct ophthalmoscopes have a white, green and blue light option. The white light is useful for general periocular examination and examination of the conjunctiva, cornea and iris. There are several lenses incorporated into this instrument and if the plus ten lens is utilized, the instrument then acts like a mini microscope.

The blue light is particularly useful for inspection of the corneal surface after instillation of fluorescein dye (see below). Like all other aspects of the examination, the anterior segment is examined in a systematic way beginning with the conjunctiva, cornea, anterior chamber (the space between the cornea and iris) and the iris, so essentially the examiner is moving gradually from the front to the back of the eye.

Certain eye drops facilitate examination of the anterior segment. The most commonly used eye drop is fluorescein which is useful at detecting abnormalities of the corneal epithelium such as corneal abrasions or dendritic ulcers caused by herpes simplex virus. Fluorescein is instilled into the inferior fornix of the eye, and the anterior segment is then examined using cobalt blue light. The chemical properties of the dye allow it fluoresce and thereby highlight epithelial defects under cobalt blue light.

Rose Bengal is a red soluble dye that is used to stain degenerate corneal epithelium and is particularly useful in the assessment of dry eye. The patient must be warned that these drops can cause extreme ocular discomfort. It is therefore advisable to instill a drop of topical anaesthetic prior to its use.

Topical anaesthetic drops can be useful if an eye is particularly painful. Instillation of topical anaesthetic can reduce discomfort and facilitate examination. The most commonly used drops are Oxybuprocaine 4% (Benoxinate), Proxymetacaine 0.5% (Ophthaine) and Tetracaine 0.5% (Amethocaine).

The Posterior Segment

The posterior segment is that part of the eye behind the iris. Posterior segment examination, outside the eye clinic, is often performed without pupillary dilation because of the risk of instigating angle closure glaucoma. The risk of missing retinal pathology by examining through an undilated pupil is significantly greater than the small risk of inducing angle closure and therefore pupil dilation is recommended.

Tropicamide 1% is the drop most commonly used to dilate the pupil. Prior to instilling any dilating drops, it is important to explain to the patient that visual blurring will occur for several hours and therefore driving is not advisable until the effects have subsided. Each type of drop will blur the vision for a certain length of time and may make some activities such as reading more difficult also. Such drops are also likely to induce photosensitivity as the normal pupil responses will be temporarily paralysed. Alternatives to tropicamide include phenylephrine 2.5% or cyclopentolate 1%

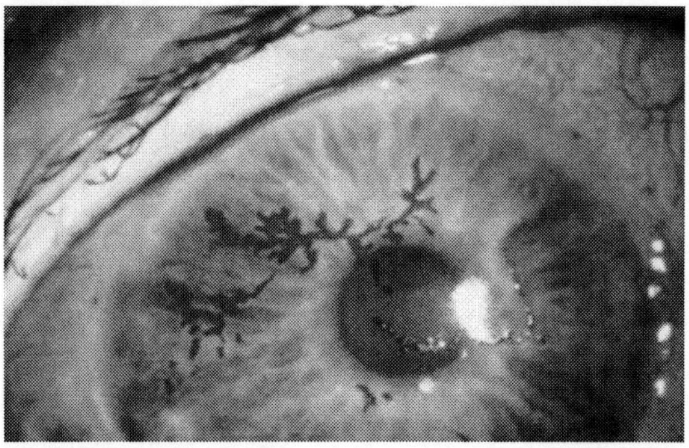

Figure 11. Rose Bengal staining of the Cornea.

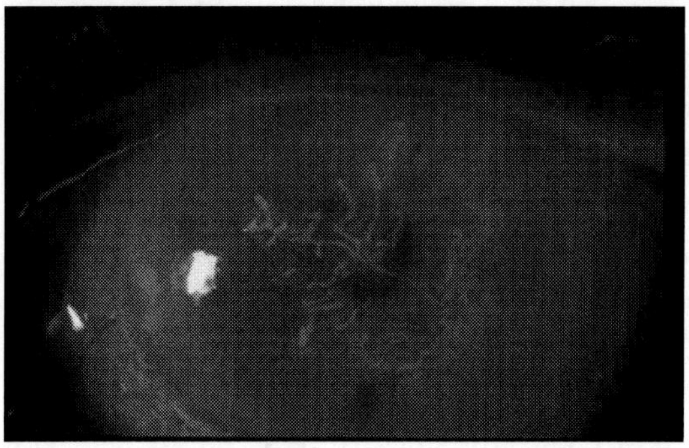

Figure 12. Fluorescein staining of a Dendritic Ulcer.

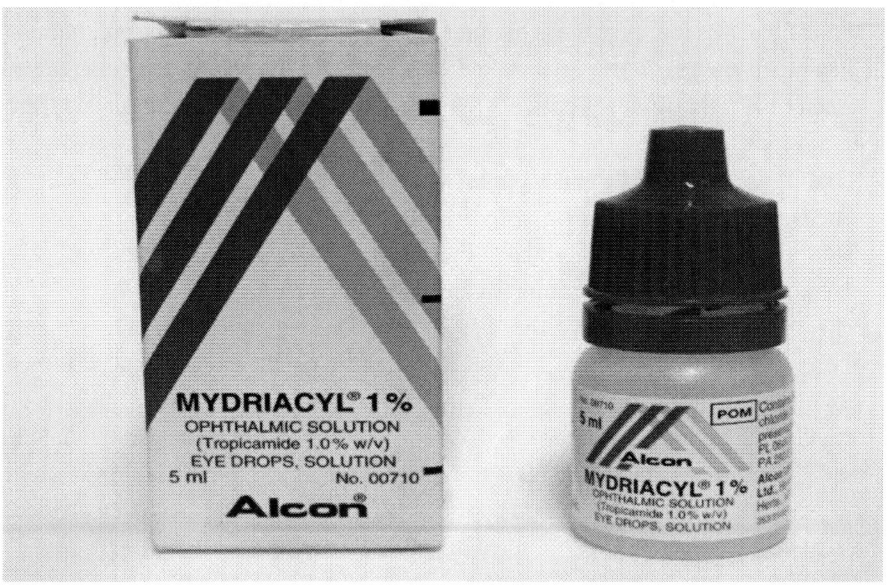

Figure 13. Tropicamide 1% dilating drops.

Drops Used to Dilate the Pupil in Ophthalmic Examination

- *Tropicamide 1%* - synthetic analogue of atropine - maximum effect 20 to 30 minutes -action up to 6 hours.
- *Phenylephrine 2.5% or 10%* - synthetic compound similar to adrenaline - maximum effect at 30 minutes - duration of action up to 5 hours - a concentration of 2.5% is preferred as systemic side effects such as hypertension can be related to the 10% preparation.
- *Cyclopentolate 0.5% or 1%* - synthetic compound to atropine - causes both mydriasis (pupil dilation) and cycloplegia (paralysis of ciliary body) -required mainly when checking young children for glasses - maximum effect 20-30 minutes - duration of action up to 24 hours - 0.5% preparations are used in children under 1 year of age.

Following instillation of a mydriatic agent, the patient is asked to wait until the pupils are sufficiently dilated. This can take longer in patients with dark irises but generally takes about twenty minutes. The posterior segment is then examined using either a direct ophthalmoscope or a slit lamp. Other techniques can be used within the setting of the eye clinic but are not relevant in this chapter. The procedure for examining the posterior segment of the eye is outlined below.

Examination of the Posterior Segment

- Check the red reflex on both sides - this is seen when light enters the pupil and is reflected from the retina.
- The examiner will be very close to the patient when examining the posterior segment - the field of view that the examiner obtains through the direct ophthalmoscope is dependent on the working distance, therefore the closer the working distance the greater the field of view - patients may find this uncomfortable if they are not warned in advance.
- Traditionally the right eye is examined first.
- The patient is asked to fixate on a distant object.
- The optic disc is first examined - documenting size, colour, presence of swelling or haemorrhage and any other abnormality.
- The vascular arcades leave the disc - there are two superiorly and two inferiorly - these are followed out to the retinal periphery in all four quadrants and any abnormalities are documented.
- Finally, the patient is asked to look directly into the light - this can be uncomfortable and therefore is deliberately left until last - the macular area is now examined and any abnormalities such as pigmentary changes, presence of exudates or bleeding are documented.

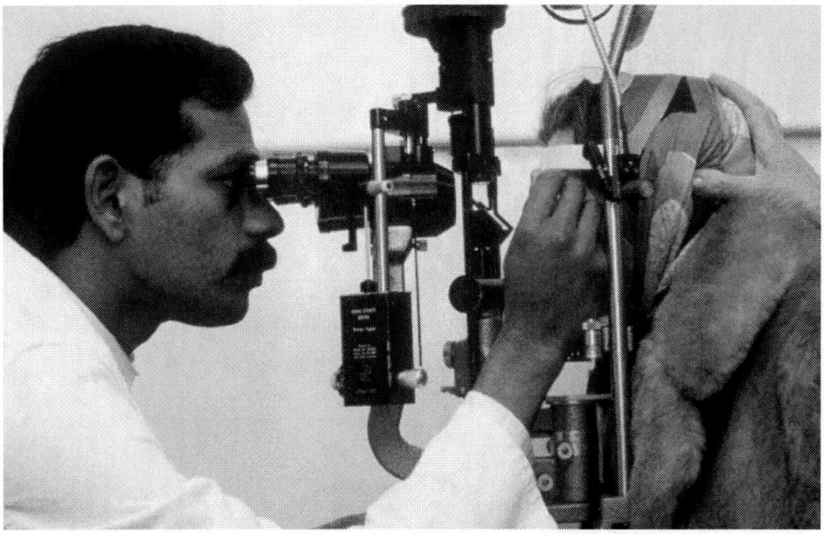

Figure 14. Examination of the Posterior Segment using Slit Lamp Biomicroscopy.

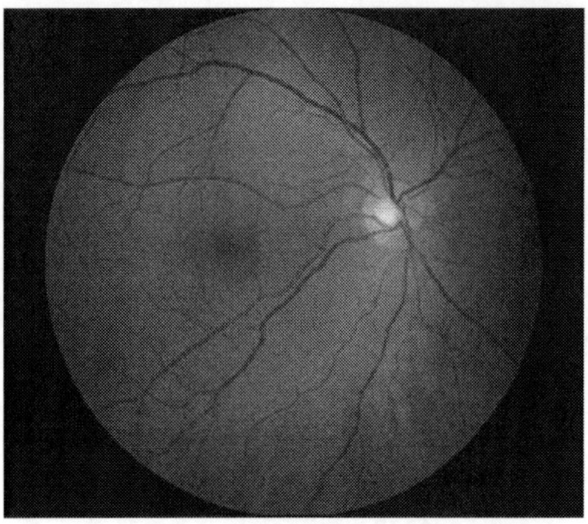

Figure 15. Normal retinal fundus.

Conclusion

The ocular history is similar to other medical histories and is undertaken in a systematic way. The eye is a particularly sensitive area of the body and this must be considered when undertaking ocular examination. A clear description of what is to take place prior to commencing the examination ensures a more endurable experience for the patient and a more rewarding and informative process for the clinician. Examination of the very old or very young may be more challenging, and the examination may therefore need to be adjusted to suit the age and ability of the patient. Clear communication in all cases and a systematic approach throughout, as outlined above, ensures the best results.

Pearls

- Listen, listen, listen – the clues are in the history.
- Look at the entire person, not just the eyes – remember lots of eye diseases have systemic manifestations, and lots of systemic diseases involve the eyes.
- Examine lots of eyes – it is only in appreciating what is normal that abnormal findings will be become obvious.
- Be able to measure visual acuity in adults and children – understand the principles of Snellen acuity and 'pin hole' or best corrected vision.
- Develop a systematic approach to examining the eye, starting from front to back.
- Life threatening problems can manifest with ocular symptoms – look at the whole patient and not just the eyes in isolation.

Pitfalls

- Don't assume that all red eyes are due to conjunctivitis – have a long list of differential diagnoses for this symptom.
- Not all conjunctivitis is of the simple bacterial variant – be suspicious of purulent, non responsive conjunctivitis in adults and children and think about the possibility of sexually transmitted infections and the need for investigation.
- Don't forget to ask about trauma – be especially cautious if a patient gives a history of hammering and consider the possibility of an intraocular foreign body.
- Don't forget about other systemic symptoms – signs in the eyes can be an indicator of problems elsewhere in the body.

Tips for the OSCE

General approach:

- As with any clinical situation, your approach to the patient is crucial. Be courteous at all times, introduce yourself properly, explain clearly what you are going to do and most importantly, listen to the patient, they often volunteer all the information that you need!

Use of Equipment:

- Become familiar with the examination techniques and especially the use of the direct ophthalmoscope - it is easy for an examiner to spot students who are turning it on for the first time!

Common Ophthalmic Complaints:

- Loss of vision, red eye, diplopia, and ocular irritation and pain are common presenting complaints to the general practitioner and the eye clinic - be familiar with the differential diagnosis, examination, investigation and management of each of these problems.

Associations between Medical Conditions and Ophthalmology

- Be aware of the relationship between medical conditions such as diabetes, rheumatoid arthritis, hypertension, multiple sclerosis, thyroid dysfunction and collagen vascular disorders and their ophthalmic manifestations.

Drug toxicity and the eye

- Several drugs used in medicine can cause complications in the eye. Be aware of the effects of drugs such as steroids, tamoxifen, amiodarone, rifabutin, vigabatrin, ethambutol and chlorpromazine.

Be prepared

- Preparation for any exam, including the OSCE, is vital. Attend some sessions in the eye clinic and eye operating theatre and practice the examination techniques frequently as outlined above. Apply a systematic approach to evaluating any problem.

There are, in truth, no specialties in medicine, since to know fully many of the most important diseases, a man must be familiar with their manifestations in many organs.

Sir William Osler

References

[1] Doshi V, Ying - Lai M *et al.* Sociodemographic, family history and lifestyle risk factors for open angle glaucoma and ocular hypertension. The Los Angeles Latino Eye Study. *Ophthalmology* 2008 Apr; 115(4): 639 – 647.

[2] Lanning B. Kline, Frank. J. Bajendas, *Neuroophthalmology Review Manual*, 6th Edition, New Jersey, USA, Slack Incorporated, 2008.

In: Learning Clinical Skills
Editors: Bridget Maher and Pat Henn
ISBN: 978-1-62100-409-7

Chapter XXI

Common Things are Common. Otitis Media

Brendan Fennessy and Gerard O'Leary

Clinical Case

A mother brings her 14-month-old son to the General Practitioner. The child has been off form for the past 24 hours with a runny nose, raised temperature, irritability and off his food. Mother gave the child oral paracetamol but the child had a restless night and remains hot and irritable.

On examination, signs of URTI are present. Temperature is 38C. Examination of the throat reveals mild pharyngitis. Lower respiratory system examination is normal. Examination of the ears using an auriscope reveals a bulging, red, tympanic membrane on the right side. There is no evidence of perforation of the tympanic membrane or fluid behind the tympanic membrane.

Diagnosis: right acute otitis media (Figure 1).

Discussion

Otitis media (middle ear infection) is an extremely common childhood disorder. Fever usually occurs and may precipitate a febrile convulsion. Ear pain (otalgia) is a key feature, and children frequently wake up very distressed having initially fallen asleep. Pain may cause infants to become restless and irritable. Loss of hearing can also occur. A discharge from the ear may occur if the eardrum has perforated. Otitis media usually has a rapid onset and follows an upper respiratory tract infection.

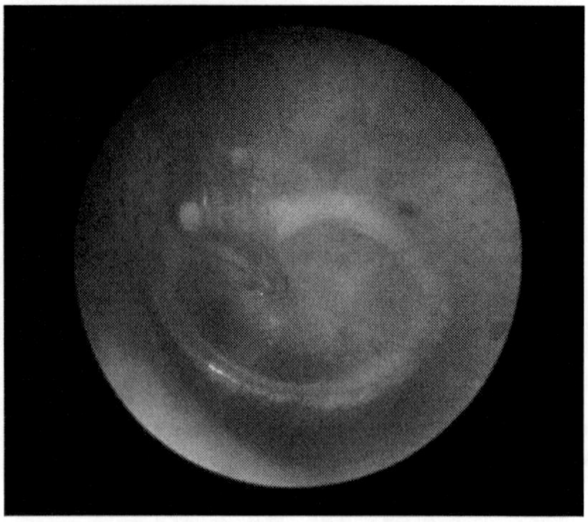

Figure 1. Otitis Media.
Author B Welleschik Copyright Permission granted under the terms of the *GNU Free Documentation License,* Version 1.2 or any later version published by the Free Software Foundation).

On examination, the tympanic membrane is inflamed and the epithelium of the membrane is often distorted ('pavement' epithelium) or bulging. There may be loss of the normal light reflex. Fluid may be seen behind the drum - otitis media with effusion (OME).

ENT History and Examination – General Principles

A comprehensive history and examination are essential in the diagnosis and treatment of Otolaryngology (ENT) conditions and, in many cases will provide a clinical diagnosis without the need for radiological or other investigations.

In taking any history, it is essential to enquire about *core symptoms* relevant to the system in question. Examples of these in ENT are the symptoms of progressive hoarseness, dysphagia or a non-healing ulcer of the tongue. This should immediately alert us to potentially serious pathology i.e. malignancy. Similarly, a child of two years with poor speech development should alert us to the possibility of a hearing loss.

The ear, nose and throat examination in many cases confirms our clinical suspicions from the history, and it is essential that the student is capable of recognizing and diagnosing common ENT clinical conditions including middle ear effusions, nasal polyps, quinsy etc.

In taking a history or performing an examination in ENT, one must consider all three areas (namely 'ear', 'nose' and 'throat') as *inter-dependent* - often all three are jointly involved in the disease process. A complete ENT history involves questioning about all three areas. A good example of this is the symptom of otalgia which may be caused by an acute ear infection, referred pain from dental infection, tonsillitis or a tonsillar cancer. This is because the tympanic membrane shares a sensory nerve supply with the upper aerodigestive tract via the V, VII, IX and X Cranial Nerves. ENT examination must include all three areas.

The finding of a middle ear effusion in an adult may result from a malignant mass in the post-nasal space obstructing the Eustachian tube leading to fluid accumulation. Thus a full ENT examination with inspection of the post-nasal space is essential if a potentially life-threatening condition is not to be missed. Attention to the above principles will ensure that the presenting symptoms will not be dealt with in isolation and enable optimal clinical management.

History

The first step is to note the *major presenting symptom.* In obtaining a history, we must *always* include name, age, presenting complaint and duration of complaint. *'Mr. Smith, is a 50 year-old-man who presents with a 7 day history of a left earache.'* The above history is then expanded and we enquire about the following symptoms in relation to presenting ear conditions.

Hearing loss	- uni/bilateral, impact on work/social activities - speech delay (children)
Otalgia	- local ear pathology- otitis media/externa - referred – dental, upper aerodigestive tract
Tinnitus	- nature, severity, unilateral/bilateral
Otorrhoea	- purulent, mucopurulent, clear
Pruritis	- dermatitis of the ear canal skin, psoriasis
Vertigo	-sensation of rotation nature: *duration,* nausea, vomiting
Facial weakness	- partial, complete
Nasal and throat symptoms	- see below.

Past medical/social/drug history must include: pregnancy/birth/neonatal problems, meningitis, grommet insertion or other ear surgery, head injury, noise exposure, drug history (chemotherapy).

Nose

The nose should not be looked at in isolation but as an entity closely linked to the paranasal sinuses and the history should ascertain the following 'sino-nasal' symptoms. With regard to sino-nasal conditions, it is particularly important to ascertain if they are perennial or seasonal problems.

- *Obstruction* - unilateral/bilateral, perennial/seasonal
- *Rhinorrhoea* - serous/mucoid, blood stained
- *Itching/sneezing* - rhinitis
- *Facial pain/pressure*- sinusitis, dental, TMJ, neuralgic
- *Epistaxis* - unilateral/ bilateral, medications, severity
- *Taste/smell function* - no taste in absence of smell (anosmia)
- *Snoring/mouth breathing* - severity, apnoea episodes
- *Eye/Visual symptoms* - epiphora, sinusitis involving the orbit
- *Ear and Throat symptoms*

Past medical history/social/drug history must enquire about previous nasal injury or surgery, aspirin sensitivity, allergies, anticoagulants, bleeding disorders etc.

Throat

The 'throat' is essentially the upper aerodigestive tract and the history must include:

- *Sore throat* - onset, associated with dysphagia, hoarseness etc.
- *Hoarseness* - inflammatory, malignant, voice abuse
- *Dysphagia* - inflammatory, neoplastic, bolus, neuromuscular, weight loss
- *Neck Lump* - midline, lateral, duration, progression
- *Stridor* - onset, severity, inspiratory, expiratory
- *Cough* - dry, productive, haemoptysis
- *Oral ulceration* - dentition
- *Otalgia*
- *Ear and Nose symptoms*

The past medical/social/drug history and social history must include *smoking history* (active, passive) and alcohol intake.

Examination

Observe for any craniofacial abnormality, facial asymmetry, obvious neck or facial swelling, mouth breathing (adenoid facies) or stridor.

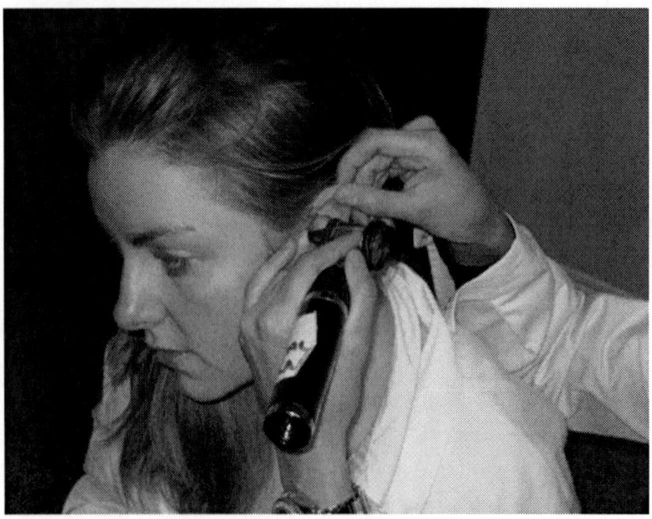

Figure 2. Ear examination.

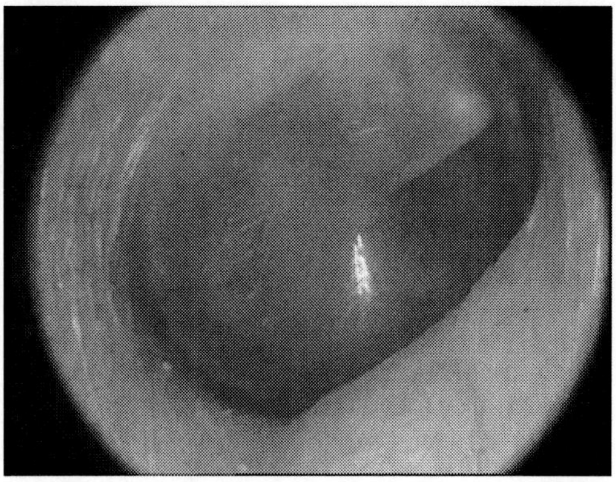

Figure 3. Normal tympanic membrane.

Ear

Look for any scars around the ear, inspect the pinna and external auditory canal. Using the biggest speculum that fits in the canal, pull the pinna gently backwards and upwards and introduce the auriscope to view the external ear canal (Figure 2) and tympanic membrane (Figure 3).

Conversational voice (CV) and whisper voice (WV) testing are a good guide to the hearing thresholds.

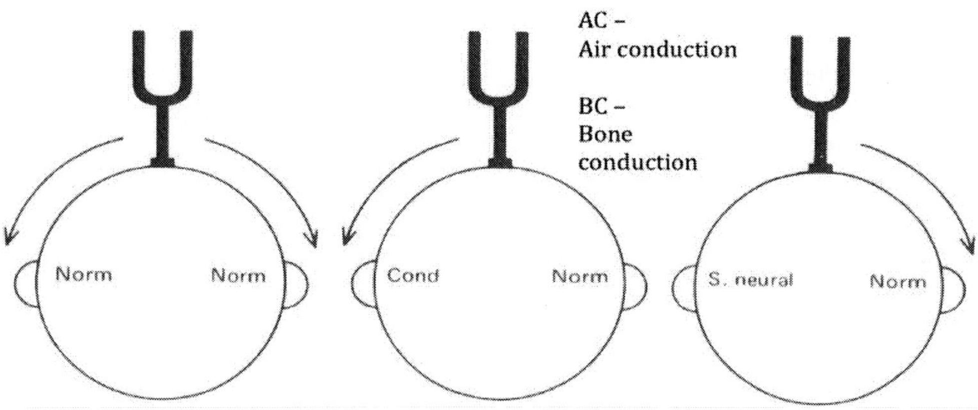

Figure 4. Weber Test.

Tuning Fork Tests

Weber

Oscillating tuning fork on the forehead (sound heard loudest on the left implies a conductive hearing loss on the left or sensorineural hearing loss on the right -Figure 4).

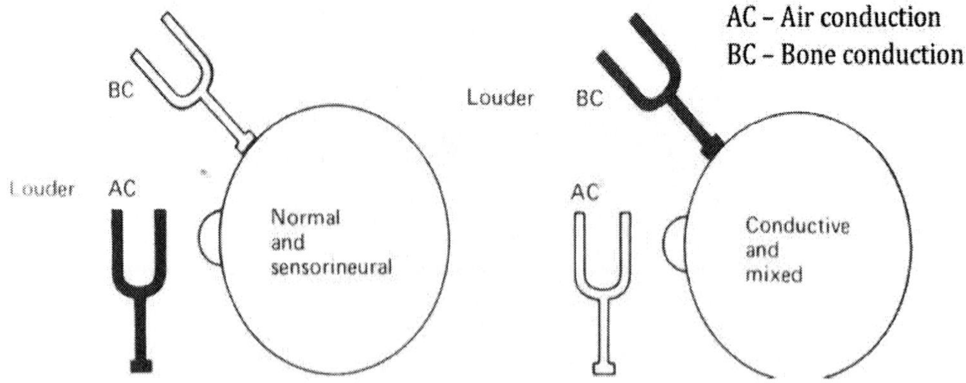

Rinne Positive: AC > BC – normal.
Rinne Negative: BC > AC - conductive loss.

Figure 5. Rinne Test.

Rinne Test

Oscillating tuning fork heard parallel to the external canal - air conduction should be louder than when placed on the mastoid postero-superior to the pinna (bone conduction). Bone conduction (BC) > air conduction (AC) implies a conductive hearing loss (Figure 4).
Cranial Nerve examination – Pay particular attention to cranial nerves VII and VIII.

Pearls

- The normal tympanic membrane appears grey and shiny and has a light reflex.
- Always examine the pinna first - check the skin for eczema – its presence indicates the possibility of otitis externa in the canal.
- Practice holding the auriscope properly (at its point of balance). Use left hand for left ear and right hand for right ear. Gently pull pinna upwards and backwards.
- In severe otitis externa or furunculosis, the external auditory meatus may be completely occluded and any attempt at otoscopy may cause severe pain.

Pitfalls

- Always examine the throat in a patient complaining of earache. Ear pain can be referred from the throat and can also be caused by tempero-mandibular joint dysfunction, herpes zoster (Ramsay Hunt Syndrome), dental disease and malignancy.
- Insert the auriscope slowly –always examine the entire canal.
- When examining infants, toddlers and young children, it is important to position the child correctly in the parent's lap. Ask the parent to sit the child sideways on their lap and to use one hand to hold the child's head against their chest and the other to hold the child's arms.

- When examining infants, toddlers and young children, hold the auriscope in the horizontal position between your thumb and index finger and middle finger. Rest your remaining two fingers (ulnar border of hand) against the side of the child's head - if the child jerks his head, your hand and the auriscope also move, preventing the ear piece of the auriscope from hitting against the meatus, external canal or eardrum and causing trauma and pain.

Tips for the OSCE

- Get plenty of practice - it is obvious who has done few and who has done many examinations!
- Explain to the patient what you are going to do.
- Always inspect and comment on the pinna.
- Wait until the child/baby is settled before attempting an examination.

Men are more apt to be mistaken in their generalizations than in their particular observations

Machivelli

Index

B

C

D

E

F

G

H

I

J

K

L

M

N

O

P

Q

R

T

U

V

W

X

Y